CANCERS
OF THE
HEAD & NECK

From Diagnosis to Treatment

Third Edition

WILLIAM M. LYDIATT, M.D.
PERRY J. JOHNSON, M.D.

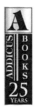

Addicus Books
Omaha, Nebraska

An Addicus Nonfiction Book

ISBN 978-1-943886-82-1
Book design and illustrations by Jack Kusler

This book is not intended to be a substitute for a physician, nor do the authors intend to give advice contrary to that of an attending physician.

Library of Congress Cataloging-in-Publication Data
Names: Lydiatt, William M., 1962- author. | Johnson, Perry J., 1964- author.
Title: Cancers of the head & neck : from diagnosis to treatment / William M. Lydiatt, MD., Perry J. Johnson, M.D.
Other titles: Cancers of the head and neck
Description: Omaha, Nebraska : Addicus Books, [2019] | Includes index.
Identifiers: LCCN 2019001935 (print) | LCCN 2019003048 (ebook) | ISBN 9781950091072 (pdf) | ISBN 9781950091096 (kdl) | ISBN 9781950091089 (epub) | ISBN 9781943886821 (paperback)
Subjects: LCSH: Head–Cancer–Popular works. | Neck–Cancer–Popular works. | BISAC: MEDICAL / Oncology. | HEALTH & FITNESS / Diseases / Cancer.
Classification: LCC RC280.H4 (ebook) | LCC RC280.H4 L93 2019 (print) | DDC 616.99/491–dc23
LC record available at https://lccn.loc.gov/2019001935

Addicus Books, Inc.
P.O. Box 45327
Omaha, Nebraska 68145
AddicusBooks.com
Printed in the United States of America
10 9 8 7 6 5 4 3 2 1

For our patients and their loved ones,
with our profound thanks for teaching us
the meaning of courage, humor, and life.

CONTENTS

Acknowledgments

We wrote this book to provide a resource for patients as they begin to grapple with their cancer diagnosis or that of a loved one. Head and neck cancers are relatively uncommon, so finding accurate and useful information can be difficult.

Hopefully, knowledge you gain from this book will reduce your anxiety and help you cope with a diagnosis and treatment. When you are better informed, you are able to ask valuable questions and you can be more involved in your treatment. As a result, you will feel more in control and can take a positive role in your own care.

We do not intend to serve as substitutes for your doctor or other health-care professionals. We do hope you will use this book as a resource whether you have cancer or are caring for someone who does. We have attempted to explain in readily understandable terms the types of cancers found in the head and neck region, treatment options, treatment side effects and ways to deal with them, and what you might expect as you work through your treatment. We have also tried to stress the importance of one's emotional health after a diagnosis of cancer and its ensuing treatment.

We are indebted to many people in the creation of this book. We thank Dr. Yungpo Bernard Su of Nebraska Cancer Specialists for his expert assistance with the chapter on chemotherapy. We thank publishers Rod Colvin and Jack Kusler of Addicus Books; they provided critical insights and expert commentary.

We owe our mentors and partners a tremendous debt of gratitude for all they have taught us. We also thank our families, who are a source of constant joy and fulfillment. Finally, we express our gratitude to our patients for helping us to see the depth of their courage and commitment.

INTRODUCTION

Cancer. Few words convey such power, fear, helplessness, anger, and sadness. Virtually all of us have been personally touched by this disease. It seems everyone has a unique reaction upon hearing this word in association with themselves or a loved one. However, because no single cancer behaves exactly the same, part of the fear associated with cancer comes from its unpredictable nature. Nowhere is this more true than with cancers affecting the mouth, throat, voice box, sinuses, thyroid, and salivary glands—collectively known as head and neck cancers. These cancers involve the most basic aspects of our humanity—our ability to speak and eat, even our appearance. Coping with these are important issues for all people with head and neck cancer.

We hope this book will help you better understand cancers of the head and neck. Hopefully, this knowledge will reduce some of your anxiety. The better informed you are, the more you can be involved in your treatment. By becoming involved, you will feel more in control and better able to take a positive role in your own care.

We have attempted to explain the types of cancers found in the head and neck region, treatment options, treatment side effects and ways to deal with them, and what you might expect as you work through your treatment. We have also tried to stress the importance of one's emotional health after a diagnosis of cancer and the treatment. By understanding more about this disease, you will be better able to formulate questions for your doctor and take a more active role in your treatment.

We wish you the best in your journey ahead. We understand the profound impact a cancer diagnosis may have on you. We hope this book will help in some small way to make it a tolerable and even life-affirming experience.

PART I

UNDERSTANDING
HEAD AND NECK CANCERS

At the Cancer Clinic

She is being helped toward the open door
that leads to the examining rooms
by two young women I take to be her sisters.
Each bends to the weight of an arm
and steps with the straight, tough bearing
of courage. At what must seem to be
a great distance, a nurse holds the door,
smiling and calling encouragement.
How patient she is in the crisp white sails
of her clothes. The sick woman
peers from under her funny knit cap
to watch each foot swing scuffing forward
and take its turn under her weight.
There is no restlessness or impatience
or anger anywhere in sight. Grace
fills the clean mold of this moment
and all the shuffling magazines grow still.

—*Ted Kooser*
Poet Laureate
of the United States
(2004–2005)

1

OVERVIEW: HEAD AND NECK CANCERS

If you have cancer of the head or neck, you are not alone. Each year, more than 60,000 Americans develop a cancer of the head or neck, which includes cancers of the lip, mouth, tongue, tonsils, throat, larynx (voice box), salivary glands, nose, and sinuses. In fact, throughout this book, we refer to "cancers of the mouth and throat," because we are typically referring to a part of the mouth or throat. Nearly 75 percent of these new cases are in men. The incidence of mouth and throat cancer among women is, however, on the rise. As many as 500,000 men and women in the United States are survivors of these cancers.

Understanding Cancer

Cancer is a group of cells growing out of control. Let's take a closer look at how this process occurs. Our cells contain a complicated set of instructions called *DNA*. These instructions tell a cell how to perform its job—that is, how to be a skin cell, a brain cell, a liver cell, and so on. They also tell the cell when to reproduce and when to die. DNA is the major part of our *chromosomes,* which determine our individual traits such as height and hair color, and even many aspects of our personality. In short, DNA is often called the "instruction manual" for life.

DNA Becomes Damaged

Sometimes, though, DNA can tear down what it has built. If a cell's DNA is damaged—for example, by a virus or toxic substance—certain instructions from the DNA will cause the cell to die. Occasionally, instead of dying, the abnormal cell will begin reproducing rapidly, creating ever greater numbers of new cells that also carry the DNA damage.

The more abnormal a cell's DNA becomes, the more abnormally the cell will behave. In turn, this abnormal behavior creates more and more mistakes within the cell. These DNA "mistakes" are called *mutations*. It appears that damaged cells must have between six and ten different mistakes before they begin behaving like a cancer.

Take, for example, the cells that make up the mucous membrane of the mouth and throat. These cells normally divide and reproduce only when old cells die or other cells are scraped away in normal activities such as chewing and swallowing. Normally, the cells next to those that have died or been scraped away will reproduce to replace them. After the dead cells have been replaced, the process of cell growth stops.

However, if the cells have become damaged when they are exposed to such things as excessive tobacco smoke, alcohol, or other hazards, they may pass the damage on to the next generation of cells as they reproduce. As larger and larger generations of abnormal cells are formed, they may eventually become visible as white or red patches in the mouth or throat. These are known as *precancerous lesions*. With time, the lesions may increase in both size and abnormality until they finally become true cancers.

How Cancer Spreads

Unfortunately, the out-of-control cell growth that causes cancer does not usually stop with the formation of a single tumor. Instead, the abnormal cells tend to invade surrounding tissue and can spread even further, through

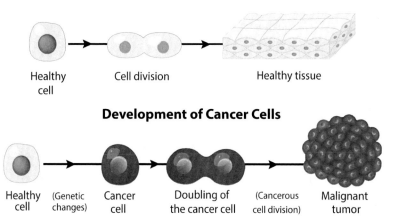

Normal Cell Development

Healthy cell → Cell division → Healthy tissue

Development of Cancer Cells

Healthy cell → (Genetic changes) → Cancer cell → Doubling of the cancer cell → (Cancerous cell division) → Malignant tumor

the blood or through the lymphatic system. The *lymphatic system* includes channels, similar to veins that carry white blood cells and nutrients and drain waste products away from tissues and cells. These channels contain rounded masses of tissue called *lymph nodes,* which filter bacteria, viruses, and cancer cells out of the lymphatic fluid.

When cancer spreads beyond the place where the first abnormal cells develop, each resulting new cancer is called a *metastasis.* When a group of cells grows into a mass that does not invade or spread elsewhere, the mass is called a *benign*—that is, a noncancerous—*tumor,* and it has a much better prognosis than cancer.

Grading Cancer

Health professionals speak of cancers in terms of "grade." Some cancers are graded as being high or low. The grade indicates how fast the cells are reproducing and may have implications in treatment. A higher grade indicates that a cancer is more aggressive, and there is a greater likelihood that the cancer will recur after treatment. Lymph node involvement is also more likely in a high-grade cancer than a low-grade cancer. And, high-

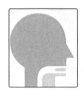

Cure rates are relatively high with cancers of the head and neck cancer. As high as 50 percent. Think positive—that you will be one of those cured.

B.L., M.D.
Surgeon

grade cancers are more likely to spread to other areas of the body. High-grade cancers are typically treated with surgery followed by radiation while low-grade tumors are often treated with surgery alone.

Causes of Head and Neck Cancer

Tobacco

Smoking cigarettes or chewing or sniffing tobacco can put a person at high risk for cancer. All forms of tobacco are dangerous, but cigarette smoke is probably the most dangerous. Most people automatically think of lung cancer when they think of the risks of smoking, but cancer can form at any site that has contact with tobacco or its by-products. In fact, 75 percent of people with mouth and throat cancer have been users of tobacco in some form.

The tissues of the mouth and throat are directly exposed to tobacco's harmful chemicals, many of which you've probably never heard of. They include such chemicals as formaldehyde, benzo(a)pyrene nitrogen oxides, urethane, nickel, cadmium, radioactive polonium, hydrazine, and N-nitrosodiethylamine. These chemicals are known to damage the inner workings of cells at the site of contact.

Tobacco products can also damage other areas of the body, including the sinuses, esophagus, salivary glands, lungs, kidneys, and bladder. All these body parts tend to be sensitive to the effects of tobacco. Damage to these more distant parts of the body occurs after special proteins called *enzymes* have broken down the chemicals in tobacco. These broken-down products of tobacco can themselves be harmful. When the kidneys and bladder, for example, come into contact with these products, cellular damage can occur in those areas as well as in the mouth or throat.

Still, not everyone who uses tobacco will develop cancer, and some who have never used it will. In general, however, tobacco use is the biggest known cause of cancers of the mouth and throat. In fact, smoking one to two packs of cigarettes a day for twenty years or more gives you a risk of mouth or throat cancer that is two to eight times greater than that of a nonsmoker. The more you smoke, the higher your risk. Women who smoke the same as men have a higher risk than men. One pack of cigarettes a day for a woman is roughly equivalent to 1.25 packs for a man.

Alcohol

The excessive use of alcoholic beverages is known to increase the risk of mouth and throat cancers—especially those at the floor of the mouth, base of the tongue, tonsils, and lower pharynx. As many as 80 percent of people with these cancers use alcohol regularly. Heavy drinking, five or more drinks per day, creates a risk that is five to eight times greater than that of a nondrinker. The combination of heavy alcohol use and tobacco use is particularly dangerous. For example, a person who consumes two packs of cigarettes and five drinks each day is about forty times more likely to get cancer than someone who does not smoke or drink. Hard liquor is thought to be riskier than beer or wine.

Viruses

Two viruses cause many head and neck cancers. One such virus, *Epstein-Barr virus (EBV)*, is best known for causing mononucleosis. This virus can also cause cancer in the back of the nose; this is called *nasopharyngeal cancer.*

Over the past twenty years, an epidemic of cancers of the tonsils and of the base of the tongue has emerged. These cancers are often associated with another viral infection caused by the *human papillomavirus (HPV).* This infection is common in individuals who have had five or more sex partners. Up to 75 to 80 percent of adult Americans have been infected with one type of HPV at some point in their lives. Keep in mind the exposure to the virus may have occurred years earlier. Many of these infections clear on their own without a person being aware that they ever had it. HPV occurs in many types. Most are considered low risk and don't cause a cancer to form. Some, those that are called *high-risk HPV,* may result in a cancer forming.

In the case of cancer caused by high-risk HPV, the virus enters the cells of the tonsil tissue, often through oral sex. The virus causes a mild infection; you may or may not have any noticeable symptoms. Most of the time, the immune system manages the infection and complete recovery occurs. However, in some cases, the DNA from a virus gets inserted into the DNA of the cell of the tonsil and slowly takes over that cell. The virus then reproduces more "copies" over time, and a cancer is formed in the tonsil tissue.

When a person develops cancer that may have started from a sexually transmitted virus, it may cause concern for the person just diagnosed and his or her partner. However, it is important to know that this virus may have been contracted many years, even decades, earlier, and, if so, the virus is no longer active and the person who had the virus is not infectious.

Other Toxins

Overexposure to numerous chemicals and hazardous substances can cause a variety of cancers. Mouth and throat cancers have been linked to mustard gas, wood dust, cadmium, leather manufacturing, exposure to iso-propyl alcohol manufacturing, nickel, and chewing betel nut, the seed of a type of palm tree.

Exposure to sunlight is also well known to increase the risk of skin cancers and lip cancer as well. Serious sunburns in childhood create risk for adult skin cancers. People with light skin and freckles, especially those of northern European descent, are at highest risk. It is important to use sun protection. Clothing that blocks the sun is best. The uses of sun-blocking agents is another method of sun protection but must be applied regularly, as indicated by the product label.

Severe stomach acid reflux can also elevate the risk of cancers of the esophagus and the lower throat. Exposure to radiation as a child also creates a risk for cancer in later years, as an adult.

Heredity

Although some cancers appear to run in some families, cancers of the mouth and throat tend to be inherited only through rare genetic syndromes.

- *Li-Fraumeni syndrome* is a mutation of a special gene that makes a protein necessary for repairing cellular damage. The mutation inhibits the repair process and therefore raises the risk of cancer.

- *Bloom's syndrome* is associated with short stature, increased sun sensitivity, immune deficiency, and a higher risk of mouth cancer, especially of the lip and tongue.

- *Fanconi anemia* is associated with abnormal skin pigmentation, growth retardation, and blood ab-normalities such as anemia, and this, too, carries an increased risk of mouth cancer.

- *Xeroderma pigmentosum* involves extreme sensitivity to sunlight and puts affected individuals at a much higher risk for lip and skin cancers.

If you or any of your relatives have any of these rare syndromes, or if members of your family have had head or neck cancer, ask your doctor about your degree of risk. He or she might advise you to talk with a genetics counselor, who could help assess whether you or your family members may be at particular risk.

Areas Affected by Head and Neck Cancers

Mouth

Technically, the mouth begins at the point where the upper and lower lips meet and it includes the gums, teeth, tongue, hard palate (roof of the mouth), floor of the mouth, and inner cheeks. If any one of them is compromised by disease, it can threaten a person's ability to breathe, eat, or speak.

Throat

The throat, which is called the *pharynx,* is composed of three parts, the *oropharynx, hypopharynx,* and *nasopharynx.* The pharynx begins in the back of the nose and extends down to the opening of the esophagus and includes the adenoids, tonsils, soft palate, back of the tongue, and lower throat.

The *oropharynx* is the middle part of the throat, behind the mouth. It includes the back third of the tongue, the soft palate, the side and back walls of the throat, the tonsils, and the *uvula,* the tissue that hangs down at the back of your throat.

The *hypopharynx* is the entrance to the esophagus, the tube that carries food to the stomach. The *nasopharynx* includes the adenoids, which are small masses of tissue that fight infection, and the eustachian tubes.

Head and Neck Anatomy

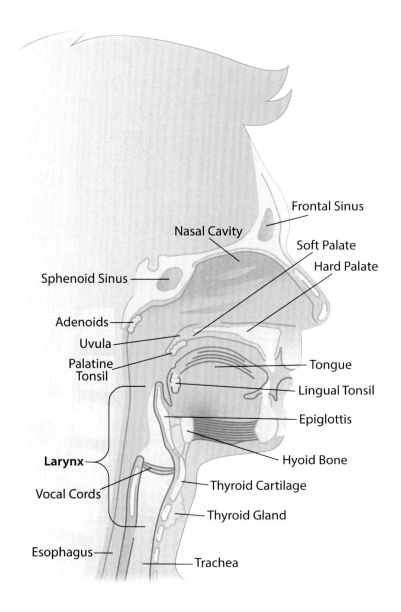

Frontal Sinus

Nasal Cavity

Soft Palate

Hard Palate

Sphenoid Sinus

Adenoids

Uvula

Palatine Tonsil

Tongue

Lingual Tonsil

Epiglottis

Larynx

Hyoid Bone

Vocal Cords

Thyroid Cartilage

Thyroid Gland

Esophagus

Trachea

The *eustachian tubes* are canals that connect the middle ear to the upper throat and the back of the nasal cavity. When fluids accumulate in the middle ear as a result of illness or infection, the eustachian tubes may become swollen or blocked. The eustachian tubes also produce the "pop" in your ears when you experience a change in altitude or air pressure.

The pharynx handles swallowing. The muscles of the pharynx squeeze food down to the esophagus, a longer tubelike structure that takes over the job until the food reaches the stomach.

Larynx

The *larynx,* or voice box, is connected to the trachea (windpipe) and is actually part of the respiratory system. It is involved in producing sound and prevents food and liquids from getting into your lungs when you swallow.

The larynx is located in front of the pharynx and just below the back of the tongue. It can be felt in the neck as the Adam's apple. It has three compartments—the *glottis, supraglottis,* and *subglottis.*

The *glottis* is formed by the *vocal cords,* which tighten and loosen to produce sounds of varying pitch. The tongue, cheeks, teeth, and lips then shape the sounds into words. Pitch variation is an important, expressive aspect of speech but a minor requirement for basic communication.

The *supraglottis,* or top portion of the voice box, consists of a flap of cartilage called the *epiglottis* and other structures called *false vocal cords,* which we use for whispering. Together, these structures push food and liquids backward, away from the trachea and into the pharynx. This prevents us from choking and keeps food and liquids out of the lungs. The *subglottis* is the space below the true vocal cords and just above the trachea.

Paranasal Sinuses

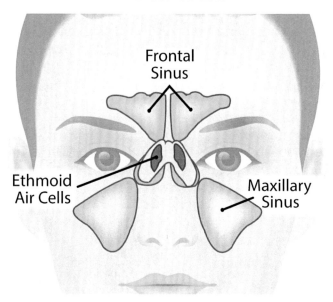

Sinuses

The *paranasal sinuses,* located behind and at the base of the nose, are air-filled cavities in the skull. These sinuses are lined with mucous membranes. Sinuses play an important role in speech—the sound made by your larynx and throat resonates in your sinuses, making your voice audible and giving it your own unique sound. When you get a cold, your sinuses become congested and the membranes swell, giving the sound of your voice a nasal quality. The four major sinuses in your head are the *frontal, maxillary, ethmoid,* and *sphenoid sinuses.*

The *frontal sinus,* located above your eyes and behind your forehead, does not develop until adolescence. It determines the shape of your adult forehead, and the thick bones surrounding it protect your brain from injury. Tumors usually do not affect the frontal sinus.

The sinuses most susceptible to tumors are the maxillary and ethmoid sinuses. The *maxillary sinuses,* located under your eyes, help form the floor of your eye sockets.

11

They are also the sinuses most frequently affected by sinus infections. Nerves that supply sensation to the middle part of your face and your top teeth run through this sinus. A tumor involving these nerves can create numbness or tingling of the face or upper teeth. Surgical removal of this sinus can also cause numbness in these areas. The *ethmoid sinuses,* containing nerves that control your sense of smell, are located between your eyes.

The bones that separate the sinuses are eggshell thin; however, they can play an important role in acting as a barrier to the spread of cancer. One such bone is the *cribriform plate,* located right on top of the ethmoid sinuses. This bone has many perforations through which the nerves for the sense of smell pass from the nose to the brain and back. Also, the *dura,* a thick covering of tissue, surrounds the brain and further inhibits the invasion of cancer cells. Still another barrier is the *periorbita,* the thick lining of the eye sockets, which protects the eyeballs from the spread of a tumor.

The *sphenoid sinus* is situated almost in the center of your head. It is surrounded by the nasopharynx below, the brain on the top and three sides, and the nasal cavity in the front. It is the least common site for sinus tumors.

Salivary Glands

The salivary glands produce *saliva,* which lubricates food for swallowing and contains special proteins called *enzymes* that begin the digestive process. There are three pairs of major salivary glands—the parotid, submandibular, and sublingual glands. The largest of these is the *parotid glands* that are located in front and beneath the ear. The *submandibular glands* are under the floor of the mouth. The *sublingual glands* lie directly under the mucous membrane covering the floor of the mouth beneath the tongue.

There are also between 600 and 1,000 minor salivary glands within the mucous membranes that line your tongue, lips, palate, throat, nose, and sinuses. These glands typically cannot be seen without magnification.

Neck
 The neck contains nerves that permit most of the activities of the mouth and throat, including the nerves to the tongue, throat, voice box, and neck muscles. If cancer invades any of these nerves, it usually destroys or damages their function. For example, if the major nerve to the tongue is invaded, you will notice a slurring of speech; and, if the nerve to a vocal cord is invaded, you will become hoarse.

 The neck also contains lymph nodes, the first areas to which mouth and throat cancers generally spread. The lymph nodes are small, bean-shaped glands that filter out bacteria, viruses, and cancer cells. They swell if they become infected or cancerous.

Types of Mouth and Throat Cancer
 The type of a cancer is determined by its cell of origin. That is, where did the cancer start—in cells of the skin, fatty tissue, muscle, cartilage, or bone? Certain areas of the mouth and throat such as the undersurface and side of the tongue and the tonsils are more prone to cancers because they come into contact with cancer-causing substances. Determining the precise type of a cancer is important because treatment will be based on the type of cancer present.

Carcinomas

Squamous Cell Carcinoma
 Squamous means "flat." Squamous cells are flat, tough, protective cells that make up the skin and also the mucous membranes inside the mouth and throat. Cancers that begin in these cells are *squamous cell carcinomas.* They represent more than 90 percent of all cancers of the

Neck Lymph Nodes

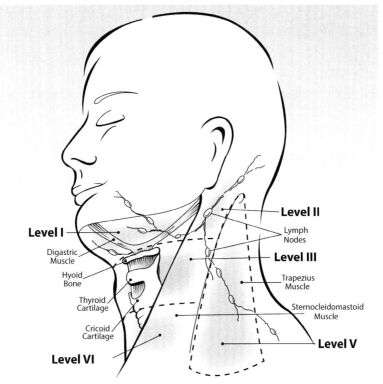

Lymph nodes in the neck are divided into five regions, shown above as levels. The lymph nodes, approximately 200 total, are located under the sternocleidomastoid muscle.

mouth and throat. They are usually caused by tobacco use or human papillomavirus (HPV). They are also one of the most common skin cancers.

Salivary Gland Tumors

More than 75 percent of tumors of the salivary glands occur in the parotid glands, located near the jaw bone and in front of the ear. Fortunately, most of these parotid growths are benign. Tumors in the submandibular glands account for about 10 to 15 percent of salivary gland tumors, but only about half of these are benign. The remaining salivary gland tumors, which occur in the sublingual and minor glands, are more often malignant. Because salivary glands contain many different types of cells, different types of cancers can arise in them. However, most are carcinomas.

Most Common Salivary Gland Cancer

The most common salivary gland cancer is *muco-epidermoid carcinoma*. It can form in any of the salivary glands, but it is seen most often in the parotid glands. In this cancer, grade is very important. Grade refers to how fast the cells are reproducing, and may have implications in treatment. For example, high-grade cancers are often treated with surgery followed by radiation, and low-grade tumors are often treated with surgery alone.

Adenoid Cystic Cancer

A common salivary gland cancer, *adenoid cystic carcinoma,* typically occurs of the minor and sublingual salivary glands (under the tongue), and possibly of the submandibular glands (under the floor of the mouth) as well. These tumors tend to grow slowly, tracking along nerves.

The weakness of a nerve, particularly a facial weakness, may indicate the presence of a adenoid cystic carcinoma. These cancers are less likely to spread to lymph nodes but many times will spread to the lungs, liver, or bones. Close, ongoing follow-up is very important. These tumors can be extremely persistent, recurring many years after treatment.

Adenocarcinoma

Adenocarcinomas arise either from minor salivary glands or from the small glands that make up the major salivary glands. Like squamous cell carcinomas, they can spread to the lymph nodes, lungs, or other organs.

Lymphoepithelial Carcinoma

This cancer occurs in the tonsils, adenoids, or at the base of the tongue, where lymph tissue is commonly found. The cancer tends to spread to lymph nodes very early and will often show up as a neck mass with a tumor in the tonsil or nasopharynx, above the roof of the mouth. These small tumors are found only after careful searching.

This is the most common cancer affecting people of Asian descent and by far the most common tumor of the nasopharynx worldwide. *Lymphoepithelial cancer* is associated with the Epstein-Barr virus, a common cause of upper-respiratory infections. The vast majority of people infected by this virus will not develop cancer, but it does seem to be associated with a high number of these cancers. Lymphoepithelial cancer is also associated with certain risk factors, including poor ventilation and a diet heavy in salted fish.

Sarcomas

These cancers can develop from the cells of muscle, fat, bone, connective tissue, or cartilage almost anywhere in the body. They are categorized either as high-grade or low-grade cancers, which helps predict their behavior and prognosis.

There are many types of sarcoma. The treatment for each depends on the site where it first arises. For example, an *osteosarcoma* may start in the bone of the upper jaw. *Rhabdomyosarcoma* begins in the muscles. This tumor is often seen in children. The most common sarcoma in adults is called *undifferentiated pleomorphic sarcoma*. It arises in the soft tissues of the head and neck. The prognosis for all sarcomas tends to depend on their size and grade. The smaller the tumor and the lower the grade, the better the prognosis.

Neuroendocrine Cancer

Melanoma
These cancers form in the cells that make pigment when they are exposed to sunlight—the cells that give you a tan. They usually occur on the skin but can also be found in all areas of the mouth and throat. This cancer can be aggressive, depending on the degree of abnormality in the cancer cells.

Esthesioneuroblastoma
This cancer begins in the olfactory nerves, which give you your sense of smell. Such a tumor can occur at any age and, in fact, is often seen in young people.

Lymphomas
Lymphomas begin in the lymph system and can occur anywhere that lymph tissue is found. The term does not refer to cancers that have originated elsewhere and spread to the lymph nodes.
Lymphomas can involve lymph nodes in one area only or throughout the entire body, including the liver, spleen, bone marrow, and even the skin. The head and neck region alone has about 200 lymph nodes. Lymphomas often arise in the neck but can also form in the tonsils, adenoids, tongue, mouth, and throat.

2

GETTING A DIAGNOSIS

Getting a cancer diagnosis can be frightening. The time one waits for various test results is stressful, to say the least. Many patients describe it as being on an "emotional roller coaster." But rest assured, cancers of the mouth and throat are among the most curable cancers if they are caught early. The survival rate for these cancers five years after diagnosis is 50 percent depending on the stage of the cancer at diagnosis. With cancers of the tongue or voice box, the rate is even higher—60 percent overall, and 90 percent if detected early. Most cancers associated with human papillomavirus (HPV) have a very high cure rate—around 70 to 90 percent.

Accordingly, it is important to get a diagnosis as soon as possible. Fortunately, with cancers of the mouth and throat, early detection is common. Why? The symptoms tend to be obvious and prompt individuals to see a physician; common symptoms include impaired tongue movement, persistent hoarseness, and a lump in the mouth or throat. If you even suspect that a change you have noticed in your body or its functions could indicate cancer, you should see a doctor without delay.

Symptoms of Head and Neck Cancers

The following symptoms should be evaluated by a physician if they persist longer than two weeks, become progressively worse, or occur on only one side of the body. In some cases, you might be referred to a specialist such as a head and neck surgeon, an oral surgeon, or an ENT physician who specializes in treating the ears, nose, and throat. An ENT physician can evaluate hearing loss, nasal obstruction, facial nerve paralysis, and hoarseness.

Hoarseness

Persistent hoarseness is one of the most common signs of cancer of the vocal cords and larynx. Sometimes it arises along with a cough, blood in the phlegm, increasingly noisy breathing, or progressive difficulty in breathing.

Sore Throat, Mouth Sore, or Lesion

A sore throat or a mouth sore that does not go away in a week or two can be a sign of throat or mouth cancer. White or red patches on the skin of the throat or mouth may be precancerous conditions known as *leukoplakia* or *erythroplakia*. They can be treated to prevent a cancer from forming. There are almost no symptoms associated with these precancerous conditions, and only a visual inspection can detect them. This is why routine evaluations by your doctor or dentist are important.

Lump in the Mouth, Throat, Neck, or Cheek

Many cancers have only one symptom at first—a lump, which is often painless. This is especially true of HPV-associated cancers and salivary gland cancers. Occasionally, people discover a mouth cancer when a lump interferes with the fit of their dentures. Any new lump should be seen by a doctor. This becomes urgent if the lump is more than half an inch in diameter, is hard and growing, and/or is located in an area where cancers are especially prone to arise, such as in the salivary gland or upper neck. Some of these lumps will be benign tumors or will be caused by infection. Lumps that are soft are rarely cancerous. Still, any new lump should be evaluated.

Change in Speech Quality

Progressive changes in speech—especially a growing inability to speak clearly or an increasingly muffled quality to your voice—could indicate tongue or throat cancer. Over time, tongue cancer can deprive a person of any ability to enunciate because it can completely restrict tongue movement. Any of the symptoms affecting speech can be accompanied by bad breath, so that, too, can be considered a possible warning sign.

Difficulty Swallowing

Cancer of the throat—either the pharynx or esophagus—can gradually make swallowing difficult. If heavier, solid foods like meat become hard to swallow at first, with lighter, softer foods and liquids increasingly presenting a problem, that could mean that a tumor is gradually narrowing the esophagus. Cancer of the pharynx may also result in a feeling that food is catching in the throat. If the lower pharynx is involved, food may get into the trachea. This is known as *aspiration,* and it generally causes coughing while eating.

Nosebleeds

If you experience recurrent nosebleeds, or if your nose is constantly plugged on one side only, you should see your doctor. These can be symptoms of a sinus or nasopharyngeal cancer blocking the nasal passage. With trauma or blowing of the nose, the tumor can crack and bleed through the nose. Most nosebleeds and nasal blockage are caused simply by dry air and a *deviated septum*—a deviation or injury to the cartilage "wall" inside the center of the nose. Other common causes include exposure to wood dust, chemicals, or other irritants.

People with a long history of nosebleeds are no more susceptible to cancer than anyone else. But nosebleeds that develop suddenly should always be investigated.

Hearing Loss and Earache

Normal hearing loss associated with aging usually occurs in both ears at about the same rate. But, if you have persistent hearing loss, a sense of fullness in one ear, or pain that is always on the same side, this may be the first sign of a tumor in the upper part of the throat (nasopharynx) that lies behind the nose. Similarly, in adults, fluid in the middle ear may indicate a tumor.

If there is no obvious cause of earache or fullness—such as allergy, viral infections, or altitude changes—the area in the upper part of the throat should be examined to rule out the possibility of a tumor blocking the *eustachian tube*—in the middle ear. The examination is performed with an instrument called a *nasal endoscope,* which allows your doctor to examine the back of your nasal passages.

In general, any earache that does not go away should be evaluated by your doctor. If the ear itself is found to be normal, with no infection, he or she will examine your throat. Persistent pain in the ear can be referred pain from an irritated nerve lower in the throat. *Referred pain* is felt in a part of the body, but the actual source of the pain is from another part of the body. For example, such pain can occur when a cancer of the throat has invaded a nerve that supplies sensation to the ear. The pain is often intensified by the act of swallowing and can be made even worse by eating hot or spicy foods. This pain is usually described as deep and penetrating. It should always be evaluated.

Facial Numbness, Asymmetry, or Changes in Eyesight

Tumors of the sinuses can damage or destroy nerves that supply sensation to the lips and cheeks. If you notice a loss of sensation in these areas, especially if you also

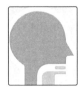

After the surgeon leaves the examining room, I make sure patients completely understand why a biopsy and the blood tests are necessary. Many patients seem reluctant to relay their fears or anxieties to the surgeon.

Rob
Nurse

have a lump or a change in your eyesight, you need to be examined. Your symptoms could be caused by a tumor of the maxillary sinus, which can push into the eye socket and put pressure on the eyeball, resulting in double vision, asymmetry, fullness of the cheek, or numbness of the cheek.

Choosing a Doctor

If you are worried about any symptoms you may be having, your best first step is to ask your family doctor to evaluate you or refer you to a specialist. After you have found an appropriate physician to evaluate your symptoms, he or she will review your medical history, discuss with you the history of your symptoms, and examine you. These steps will determine which tests come next. The following information will help you understand what happens during this first visit to a physician.

Medical History

Your medical history is likely to give your doctor a good deal of information about your susceptibility to particular kinds of cancer. You will be asked when you first noticed the problem and how it affects your life. Your doctor will also ask you about symptoms—when they started, how long they have been present, and whether they are getting worse. Even though you may have already given one doctor these descriptions, telling your story again to the next doctor will help each physician to better understand how your symptoms may be affecting you.

Repeating the story may also prompt you to remember additional details. Identifying the body parts that are affected helps to predict what kind of cancer might be present. For example, a lump that has been present for ten years with no change is not likely to be cancerous.

General Health and Medications

During your initial examination, your doctor will ask about your general health, any medications you are taking, and whether you are having any other health problems. This is important for several reasons. It will give your doctor a better idea of how much at risk you are for cancer and whether your symptoms might be caused by medications that can cause side effects such as mouth sores, plugged ears, or various kinds of pain.

Your doctor will probably ask you detailed questions about all aspects of your life, including your use of tobacco or alcohol. Such questions may make you uncomfortable at first, but they are *not* meant to invade your privacy. In fact, if your doctor does not ask such questions, he or she might miss opportunities to help you in important ways.

Physical Examination

During your physical examination, your doctor will examine your ears, nose, throat, and mouth. He or she will also check for lumps in your neck, cheeks, and thyroid gland. The doctor may use a mirror to look at your larynx and upper throat.

If a more detailed examination of your nasal passages or larynx is required, the doctor will use either a flexible or a rigid scope, inserting it after applying a topical anesthetic to numb your nose. The anesthetic does not taste good, but it eases discomfort involved in inserting the scope, which takes only a minute or two. Your doctor will then ask you to say "e," which makes your vocal cords move and identifies any abnormalities in the function of the larynx. The scope gives your doctor an excellent view of

23

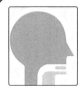

Everything seems to stop when you are diagnosed with cancer. Your world is in turmoil. I researched my cancer. I asked questions. I relied on my family and doctors, and by being actively involved, I was able to keep some control and dignity.

Jim, 58
Cancer survivor

the nasal passages and larynx, along with any lumps or ulcers that are otherwise hard to see.

Altogether, your medical history review, symptom review, and physical examination will take fifteen to thirty minutes. Some of the information will be gathered in advance by the nurse or by a questionnaire given to you in the waiting room. Make sure to answer all questions completely and truthfully. This saves time and allows you to think about any symptoms you might not have mentioned, perhaps thinking they were not relevant or not very serious. Together, the questionnaire and examination will give your doctor enough information to develop a plan, which could require tests such as those described below.

Biopsy

If your physical examination turns up a lump or ulceration, the next step is likely a biopsy. In this procedure a small sample of affected tissue is removed and then sent to a laboratory to be analyzed for cancer cells. Sometimes the tissue sample can be taken in the doctor's office—as in the case of visible sores in the mouth or using a flexible scope with special biopsy forceps. Sometimes, the biopsy requires admission to the hospital or a visit to an outpatient surgical center. During an office procedure, the sore or other affected site is numbed, and a small piece of tissue is cut out and sent out for analysis.

Certain suspicious lumps—for example, in the neck, thyroid or salivary glands—can be biopsied in the doctor's office using a procedure called *fine needle aspiration (FNA)*. Your doctor may perform or obtain an ultrasound of the neck to further investigate the lump. If a biopsy is needed, the ultrasound is often used to assist in the biopsy. In this case, your doctor can insert a very narrow needle to withdraw a sample of cells directly from the lump using the ultrasound to guide where the needle is placed. First the area is numbed with lidocaine. Usually, it takes three to five aspirations to gather enough cells for a diagnosis.

In other cases, when a biopsy cannot be taken easily in the office, your doctor may recommend that it be carried out under general anesthesia. This is a common procedure for areas like the throat and larynx, which are not as accessible as the mouth or neck. This kind of biopsy, usually performed on an outpatient basis, requires a special scope. This scope allows biopsy forceps to be inserted through it. You will almost always go home the same day a biopsy is performed.

If your symptoms suggest that you might have cancer in more than one location, your doctor might also look at your lungs or esophagus during a biopsy of throat or larynx tissue. While you are under anesthesia, he or she can feel any tumor or lesion to determine the extent of the disease without causing you pain.

Regardless of how a biopsy is performed, once the tissue sample is in the laboratory, a *pathologist* (a doctor who specializes in interpreting cell changes caused by disease) will examine the specimen under the microscope. If cancerous cells are detected, the pathologist will determine which type of cancer is present and will inform your doctor. If the initial biopsy doesn't yield enough information for an exact diagnosis, further biopsies will be needed. Biopsy results are usually back in one to five days.

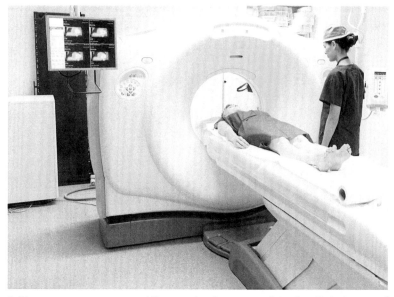

A CT scan uses computer and X-ray technology to produce detailed pictures of internal organs, bones, and tissues. Used for diagnostic purposes, a CT scan is painless.

Imaging Studies

Imaging, the general term for X-rays and body scans, is not always necessary but is commonly used. A special X-ray—a *panorex X-ray*—shows the jaw and teeth in detail and can often detect whether a cancer has invaded nearby bone. X-rays alone do not usually provide sufficient detail to evaluate masses in the mouth or throat. However, other diagnostic tests provide clear images of any suspicious lumps or lesions that can't be seen directly.

CT Scan

Computed tomography, or a *CT scan,* is an imaging tool that provides remarkable detail, showing not only what a suspicious lump looks like but how it affects surrounding tissues and whether other lumps or lymph nodes are abnormal. A chest CT scan may also be performed to evaluate whether you have any abnormalities in your lungs. A CT scan requires that you lie on a table while a tubelike machine moves over the part of the body being examined.

Usually, a CT scan involves the injection of a special solution, called *contrast,* given through a vein; this solution highlights physical structures, such as blood vessels, so that all parts of the image can easily be distinguished. The contrast feels hot when it goes into your vein.

Tell your doctor if you have a known allergy to such a contrast, are allergic to iodine, or have any kidney problems. Allergic reactions to the CT contrast are uncommon, but in cases where they might occur, either the contrast will not be used or medications or fluid will be given before the CT to minimize any ill effects. The test takes about ten to twenty minutes to administer, depending on how many areas are being examined.

MRI

Magnetic resonance imaging (MRI) is similar to a CT scan, but it is better at providing a view of internal soft tissues. For this test, you are also given a contrast solution and your body passes through a tubelike machine. During this test, you may hear loud clanging noises made by the MRI machine. These sounds are normal and should not cause you any concern. This examination takes longer than a CT and may be performed in a narrower tube.

Ultrasound Examination

Another imaging technique, *ultrasound,* is similar to the procedure doctors use to view a baby in a mother's womb. This procedure uses sound waves that transmit an image of the body part being examined onto a television monitor. The doctor or technician uses an instrument called a *transducer* to create the sound waves. The procedure is painless, and it provides detail of the thyroid, lymph nodes, and salivary glands and is often done in the doctor's office. The ultrasound does not show details of the bone or deep structures of the neck as well as CT or MRI. Ultrasound is also commonly used to help a doctor guide a needle during a biopsy.

PET Scan

A *positron-emission tomography (PET) scan* is often used to detect cancer in various parts of the body. This scan relies on a sugar contrasting agent (solution) that you are asked to drink. In PET scans, the contrast agent shows cellular activity, especially areas of increased metabolism. Cancer cells, which thrive on sugar, show up as bright areas on the scan. PET scans are typically used when the cancer involves lymph nodes.

After a Diagnosis

Part of getting a diagnosis involves the staging of cancer, which is covered in the next chapter. Doctors who treat cancer will want to determine whether the cancer has spread to nearby tissue or to more distant parts of the body.

3

STAGING CANCER

As soon as a cancer diagnosis is confirmed, the next step is to determine how advanced the disease is and whether it has spread from its original site. This is called *staging the cancer,* and knowing the stage of the cancer is essential in determining the most effective treatment. For example, is surgery the best treatment? Or will other forms of treatment, such as radiation therapy or chemotherapy, be recommended?

Staging Squamous Cell Carcinoma

The standard method of staging mouth and throat cancers is the *TNM system.* It documents the stage of the disease according to the size and extent of the original tumor and whether it has spread to other parts of the body. This worldwide system tells any health-care professional involved with your case how extensive your cancer is. It stages squamous cell carcinoma very well, and most mouth and throat cancers are of this type. Other types of cancers, including lymphoma and sarcoma, are staged slightly differently, because they behave differently from squamous cell carcinoma.

T: Size or Extent of Tumor

Each component of the TNM system is measured on a scale of 0 to 4. The "T" refers to a tumor's size or extent. *Extent* refers to how much of the original site a tumor

---

Treating Head and Neck Cancer by Stage

The TNM cancer staging system was developed to evaluate three primary factors related to treating cancer:

- Tumor **(T)** refers to the size of the primary tumor and to any tissues in the oral cavity and oropharynx where the cancer has spread.

- Node **(N)** describes the involvement of lymph nodes near the primary tumor. Lymph nodes are small, bean-shaped clusters of immune system cells that are key to fighting infections and are usually one of the first sites in the body to which cancer spreads.

- Metastasis **(M)** indicates whether the cancer has spread *(metastasized)* to other areas of the body. With oral cancer, the most common site of metastases is the lungs, followed by the liver and bones.

During the head and neck cancer staging process, your doctor will assign **T, N,** and **M** values to your cancer based on its microscopic appearance. Your doctor will review your medical history, family history, and other factors to develop an individualized treatment plan for you.

---

has invaded and whether it interferes with normal body function at that site. The T category starts at 1 for the smallest tumors and for those that impair function the least or affect the smallest area.

Some tumors are given a T category according to size, others according to extent. For example, tumors of the mouth, oropharynx, and salivary glands are easy to see and to examine physically, so they are determined only by size in two-centimeter increments, from T1 for the smallest to T4 for the largest. Tumors that are located in areas that are difficult to see or feel are graded by extent rather than size. These include tumors of the *larynx, hypopharynx, nasopharynx,* and *paranasal sinuses.* In these cases, T1 indicates the least extensive (or invasive) tumors—those that affect only a part of the original site and do not interfere significantly with body function. A somewhat more extensive tumor (one that involves all or

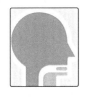

When my doctor told me that I had cancer of the throat, I thought I was going to die. I did not realize that there are different stages of the cancer. Fortunately, my cancer was small and at an early stage and I had an excellent prognosis.

Henry, 73
Cancer patient

most of the original site and either extends to an adjacent site or noticeably impedes function) is a T2.

It becomes a T3 if it has invaded the entire original site and involves additional surrounding sites or significantly hampers normal function (for example, by paralyzing a vocal cord). As soon as it moves aggressively into nearby major structures (such as the brain, in cancers of the paranasal sinuses and nasopharynx; or the thyroid cartilage, in cancers of the larynx or hypopharynx) it becomes a T4.

N: Lymph Node Involvement

The "N" category in the TNM cancer classification refers to the lymph nodes nearest the primary site, known as the *regional lymph nodes.* These are the areas to which a cancer is most likely to first spread. In the case of mouth and throat cancers, the nearest lymph nodes are in the neck. If other lymph nodes elsewhere in the body are affected by the cancer, that represents a metastasis and is reflected in the M category.

An N category is determined by the number, side of the neck, and size of affected lymph nodes found. The larger the number of affected nodes, and the larger the individual nodes, the greater the degree of involvement. A score of N0 indicates that no cancer has been detected in any of the nodes. The N score rises from 1 through 3 as more and larger cancerous nodes are discovered.

When physical examination locates lymph nodes that are larger or harder than normal, it is often difficult to tell for sure whether tumors are present or the nodes are infected by a bacterium or virus or whether cancer is present. Sometimes a biopsy is required for a firm diagnosis.

M: Spread to Other Body Sites

The "M" in the TNM system stands for *metastasis,* the spread of the cancer to other tissues, bones, or organs such as the lungs or liver. The presence of spreading cancer is suggested by blood tests or imaging techniques and confirmed by a biopsy and tissue analysis. If the cancer has not spread beyond the original site or the lymph nodes, it is designated M0. If it has spread, it is classified as M1.

Overall Stage

Once a score has been assigned to each of the three TNM components, the scores are combined to tell physicians which overall stage the cancer has reached—stage I, II, III, or IV. For example, an overall score of T1N0M0 would indicate that your tumor is of the smallest size or extent (T1), that it does not involve the lymph nodes (N0), and that it has not spread to other parts of the body (M0). This is a stage I cancer. Following is a general description of the stages:

- *Stage I* cancer is small and found only in the original site.
- *Stage II* cancer is slightly larger or more extensive but has not spread to the nearby lymph nodes or elsewhere in the body.
- *Stage III* cancer is characterized by one relatively small lymph node being involved and/or by the spread of the cancer to nearby structures or tissue.
- *Stage IV* cancer is extensive at the primary site, has extensively invaded the lymph nodes, or has metastasized to other parts of the body.

As of January 2018, cancers of the tonsils or base of the tongue that are associated with the human papillomavirus (HPV) are staged somewhat differently from the staging for cancers of the mouth, sinuses, salivary glands, skin, or voice box. If you have a cancer of the tonsil or base of tongue, a test called *p16* will be done on your biopsy specimen. If it is positive, this indicates the cancer is likely associated with HPV.

Staging Cancer in HPV Oropharynx Cancers

- *Stage I* cancer is 4 centimeters (just under 1.5 inches) or less in size at the primary site. The stage may or may not have lymph nodes involved; however, if lymph nodes are involved, they will be on the same side of the neck as the primary cancer. None of the nodes will be larger than 6 centimeters (just under two inches).

- *Stage II* cancer is either a larger primary cancer (4 cm to 6 cm) or any size tumor up to 6 cm with lymph nodes positive on both sides of the neck.

- *Stage III* cancer means an extensive primary tumor or lymph nodes larger than 6 centimeters.

- *Stage IV* cancer means it has spread to other parts of the body (M1).

Staging Lymphomas

Some kinds of cancer, because of their nature, cannot be staged with the TNM system at all, or require both the TNM system and another staging method. Lymphoma is one such cancer.

A *lymphoma* is a cancer that develops in the lymphatic system, which is located throughout the body. There are two major types of lymphoma: *Hodgkin's disease* and *non-Hodgkin's lymphoma*. Both can arise simultaneously in several sites within the lymphatic system, and so they are staged, as follows, by the number of such primary sites:

- *Stage I* is isolated to one area.
- *Stage II* appears in two locations on the same side of the diaphragm, the muscle that separates the chest from the abdomen.
- *Stage III* either involves the lymph nodes, in addition to the original lymphatic sites, or minimally involves other organs on both sides of the diaphragm (but not those that characterize stage IV).
- *Stage IV* has spread to the bone marrow, spleen, liver, or other parts of the body.

In general, the more cancerous sites there are, the more difficult it is to cure the disease. This is also true when symptoms such as fever, chills, night sweats, and weight loss are present. The presence or absence of these symptoms are therefore included in the staging designations for lymphoma (A–not present; B–present). For example, stage IA would indicate a lymphoma in only one location, with no fever, chills, night sweats, or weight loss.

Staging Sarcomas

Sarcomas, likewise, can arise almost anywhere in the body—in cartilage, muscle, bone, fat, or connective tissue. They are staged by the TNM system as well as by the grade determined by a pathologist. Why? Sarcomas usually do not spread to lymph nodes, and size is not quite as critical as in squamous cell carcinoma. The staging system for sarcomas is as follows:

- *Stage I* is a low-grade (slow-growing) tumor without lymph nodes involved.
- *Stage II* is a large (T2: greater than 5 centimeters), low-grade tumor or a small (T1), high-grade (fast-growing) tumor.
- *Stage III* is a large, high-grade tumor or any lymph node involvement.

- *Stage IV* involves spread to other parts of the body (M1).

After a Diagnosis and Staging

Depending on your diagnosis and staging of the cancer, you may be referred to a specialist, or even a team of specialists. Treating cancer often involves treatment by more than one specialist. Such a team approach offers the most comprehensive care using the skills of each specialist.

To better understand the team approach, take the example of a mouth cancer that has spread to a portion of the tongue and jaw bone. Your doctors must determine which kind of therapy will give you the best results with the fewest complications.

The decision may involve a surgeon who specializes in mouth and throat cancers, a reconstructive surgeon, a radiation oncologist, a specialist in chemotherapy, a radiologist (a specialist in X-ray and other imaging techniques), and a pathologist (a doctor who studies tissue samples in a lab to identify diseases).

If your doctors recommend surgery or radiation in or near your mouth, you will also need to be seen by a dental specialist to evaluate potential damages to your teeth. If you have cancer in your mouth or throat, you will benefit from the services of a speech therapist, before, during, or after your treatment.

Usually, the head and neck surgeon will head up your team. The team leader will serve as your primary contact during both treatment and follow-up. Your primary doctor, or family physician, will continue to serve as the point person for your overall health care.

It is also important to stress that it is perfectly reasonable for a patient to seek a second opinion if he or she has any doubts about a diagnosis or if questions are unanswered. Physicians do not find this practice unusual or inappropriate.

Determining Prognosis

A cancer's stage—how far it has advanced—largely determines the prognosis, or expected outcome, of treatment. The prognosis is usually stated as the likelihood that a person with cancer will survive five or more years after diagnosis. However, a prognosis is always a generalization. The effects of cancer vary among people—not all cases are the same.

How Soon Does Treatment Start?

As you look toward treatment, keep in mind that treatment for these cancers is considered urgent, but not an emergency. Accordingly, a general time frame for having surgery or beginning other treatment is one to four weeks after diagnosis.

Many mouth and throat cancers develop near the teeth, which can be damaged or weakened by some therapies. Therefore, it is important to have any necessary dental work taken care of before you begin cancer treatment. This includes crowns, fillings, cleaning, even extractions of non-salvageable teeth.

Your underlying health and your emotional state will also be factors in determining your treatment. The goal of your doctors is to deliver the best possible treatment so that you live the best life possible, both physically and emotionally.

Depression is a significant problem that occurs in up to 40 percent of people going through radiation treatment for head and neck cancer. Ask your doctor to explain different methods for detecting and combating depression. Many of these are discussed in chapter 9. In addition to those strategies, your doctor may recommend taking an antidepressant at the start of your treatment even if you are not currently depressed.

PART II

TREATMENT OPTIONS

Clear and Thirty-Four Degrees at 6:00 A.M. December 15

An old moon, lying akilter
among a few pale stars,
and so quiet on the road
I can hear every bone in my body
hefting some part of me
over its shoulder. Behind me,
my shadow stifles a cough
as it tries to keep up,
for I have set out fast and hard
against this silence,
filling my lungs with hope
on this, my granddaughter's
birthday, her first, and the day
of my quarterly cancer tests.

—*Ted Kooser*
Poet Laureate
of the United States
(2004–2005)

4

Surgery

Doctors perform cancer surgery with the intent of removing all the cancer they can see and feel at the time of the operation. They plan for the surgery based on physical examinations, X-rays, and scans. Most mouth and throat tumors can be treated surgically. In fact, because early detection is so common with these cancers, only 2 to 3 percent of tumors are found to be inoperable when patients are first diagnosed. Later on, some patients, approximately 15 percent, may experience metastasis to other sites in the body.

In some parts of the body, such as the mouth, surgery is usually the preferred treatment. In others, such as in the nasopharynx, surgery is seldom appropriate. The key to the decision is whether the cancer can be removed without a substantial loss of function. Surgeons with specialized training in head and neck surgery make such decisions based on the type of cancer, characteristics of the tumor, and its location.

Preparation for Surgery

Usually, you will be asked to report to the hospital about two hours before your surgery, and you'll then be taken to the preoperative area. There, you will change into a hospital gown, and nurses will start an *intravenous line,* or *IV,* to administer medication that will help you

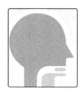

Technical advances that we have made in reconstruction of patients with cancer is amazing. I try to reassure patients, and to explain in simple terms, how we do will do their surgery.

R.J.
Plastic surgeon

relax. You may also be given medications to help reduce postoperative pain. Also, your surgeon will see you to see if you have questions or concerns.

From this point, you will be taken to the operating room. If you are still awake, you will see a machine that will monitor your heart rate and breathing. You will also see a ventilator (to help with breathing) next to the operating table. Bright lights shine overhead as the surgeons, nurses, and anesthesiologists prepare for your surgery. The operating room is sometimes rather chilly. You will be covered with a warm blanket to make you more comfortable.

After you have been moved onto the operating table, the anesthesiologist or nurse will place an oxygen mask over your mouth and nose to keep your blood rich with oxygen while you are receiving anesthesia. He or she will then administer an anesthetic through your IV tube. You might feel a mild burning sensation in your arm as the medicine enters your bloodstream. When you next awake, your operation will be over.

While you are in the operating room, your family and friends will likely be waiting in a surgery waiting room. In many hospitals, a nurse from the operating room will keep family members updated on the progress of the operation. After the operation is complete, the surgeon will meet with family and friends to inform them about the surgery.

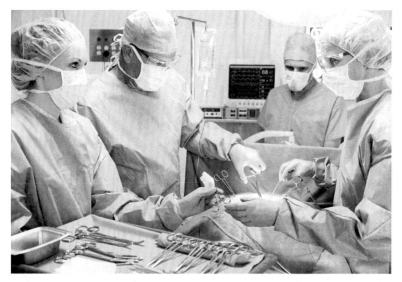

Surgery is the first line of treatement for most head and neck cancers. When a tumor is removed, surrounding tissues, called a "margin," are also removed to make sure no cancer cells remain.

Removal of a Primary Cancer

Cancer surgery involves removing the tumor and surrounding normal tissue. During the actual operation, a pathologist examines the surrounding normal tissue microscopically to see if it contains cancer cells. This process is called "doing frozen sections." The pathologist actually freezes the piece of tissue so it can be cut into extremely thin sections and examined under the microscope. If they do not show any cancer cells, it's an indication that all the cancer was removed—the "surgical margins" are considered clear of cancer. If cancer cells are detected in the surrounding tissues, more tissue is removed during the operation.

Removal of Lymph Nodes in the Neck

Most cancers beginning in the mouth or throat will spread first to the lymph nodes in the neck. If any nodes are diagnosed as cancerous they will be treated at the same time as the primary site. The removal of affected lymph nodes is called a *therapeutic neck dissection*. Sometimes, no lymph node involvement is found before the primary surgery; however, if a surgeon believes there is chance that cancer could be detected in the lymph nodes, he or she will recommend removing the nodes during the operation. The nodes will then be tested for cancer. This procedure is known as an *elective lymph node dissection,* and it carries a lower risk of complications than removing enlarged nodes in a therapeutic neck dissection.

Because of its being close to the lymph nodes in the upper neck, the salivary gland below the floor of the mouth is usually removed along with the lymph nodes in a procedure called a *selective neck dissection.* This salivary gland produces only a small portion of saliva, and a person can function without it. This operation removes the lymph nodes and fatty tissue in the neck. Occasionally, in addition, the spinal accessory nerve (which helps in raising the shoulder) is either damaged during surgery or is removed because the cancer has spread to it. If it is removed or damaged, this may lead to difficulty raising one's arm above the head. Physical therapy will usually be prescribed to help reduce the weakness and disability.

Cancer that has spread further through the neck area, into certain muscles or veins, requires a *radical neck dissection;* during this procedure, cancerous tissue is removed along with a muscle in the neck, the internal jugular vein, and the spinal accessory nerve. This operation leaves a more significant deficit in the neck.

A list of mouth and throat surgeries appears in the Appendix in the back of this book.

Side Effects of Surgery

Side effects after surgery are normal and to be expected. Not everyone experiences all side effects in the same way, but some side effects are to be expected.

Tracheostomy

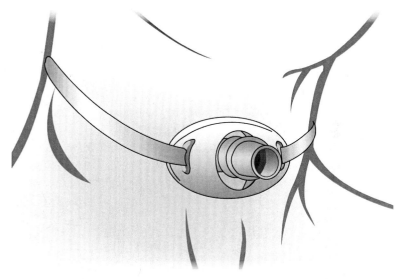

Sometimes after surgery, temporary swelling in the throat makes breathing difficult. A tracheostomy tube may be inserted into the airway.

Pain

It is common to have pain after surgery. The amount of pain depends on several factors, such as where on the body the surgery was performed, the size of the incision, and the amount of tissue removed. Medical staff has a variety of methods for managing postsurgical pain. (*See* chapter 8 for more information on postsurgical pain.)

Swelling

Swelling of the mouth or throat after surgery is common and may increase in the first two to three days but will then decrease with time. Generally this will not be an issue but on occasion swelling may lead to difficult breathing. To relieve this difficulty, a breathing tube may be inserted in the lower neck. To place such a tube, a small incision is made in the lower neck, just below the Adam's apple, to create an opening to the trachea (windpipe). A curved, hollow tube is then inserted through the opening and into the windpipe, bypassing the swelling and allowing you to breathe easily. The opening is called a *tracheostomy;* the tube is called a *tracheostomy tube.*

If your surgeons believe postoperative swelling is likely, they will perform a tracheostomy during surgery. If not, it can be done later, under a local anesthetic. In either case, a tracheostomy is almost always temporary. After the swelling is resolved—usually three to seven days after the operation—the tube is painlessly removed and the incision closes naturally in seven to ten days.

Nausea
Nausea is a common, uncomfortable side effect of the drugs used during surgery, but such side effects usually pass in twelve to twenty-four hours. The sooner you can get up and walk, the sooner the nausea will go away.

Impaired Speech
If you do need a tracheostomy tube, it might not be possible for you to speak while it is in place. The tube goes below your vocal cords and diverts the air needed for speech away from the vocal cords. If you plug the tube with your finger, this will force air up through your vocal cords and allow you to speak. Medical staff will give you instructions.

If you are temporarily unable to speak, you will be able to communicate by writing, gesturing, or pointing to special lists of common questions and phrases such as "I need to go to the bathroom." After the tracheostomy tube is removed, you will be able to speak normally again.

Lack of Appetite and Difficulty Eating
Postsurgical swelling can also make swallowing and eating difficult or impossible. For several days or a week, until any sutures in your mouth and throat are healed, you

---

Robotic Surgery

Operations that remove cancers from deep in the mouth, pharynx, or larynx may require large incisions through the muscles that control swallowing. One way surgeons avoid making such incisions is by using a special device called a *surgical robot.* The robot provides the surgeon with access to the tumor through the mouth without having to make a cut through the throat. This results in less pain and fewer swallowing difficulties for the patient.

To use this operating technique, the surgeon sits at a console and operates scopes and instruments that are inserted through the mouth. The arms of the robot have special "joints" that allow them to work around corners so they can reach areas deep in the throat.

---

might receive your nutrition through a *nasogastric (NG) tube,* which runs through your nose to your esophagus and then into your stomach. In most cases, after swelling has improved and you are able to swallow, the tube will be removed at your bedside. You will be able to begin eating again.

In some patients, however, the swelling and results of surgery make eating difficult for a longer period of time. Swelling disrupts the normal rhythm of the swallowing process that propels food down into the stomach. Also, if there is significant swelling, the tongue may not move easily. It can take time to overcome some of these difficulties and relearn to swallow. Meanwhile, a *gastrostomy (G) tube* can be placed directly into the stomach to bypass the need for swallowing. This is much more convenient than an NG tube, which interferes with speech. You or your family members will be taught how to give liquid feedings through the G tube.

Weakness

It is also common to feel very tired after surgery. This feeling will likely linger for several days. The fatigue is partially due the anesthesia used for the operation. Stress and loss of appetite contribute to this fatigue. As you recover, you will gain strength gradually.

Infection

Medical staff will take every precaution, including the use of antibiotics, to prevent infection after surgery. However, infection at the incision site may occur. Signs of infection include redness of the skin, warmth, pain, and drainage from the incision. Report such signs to your doctor immediately.

After Your Operation

Immediately after your surgery, you will be transferred to a recovery room until you awaken from the anesthesia. Then, you will be transferred to a surgical ward or, occasionally, to the intensive care unit, depending on the extent of your surgery and your overall health. You might not be fully awake or aware of what is happening during this time. You will be carefully monitored until the medical staff deems you are ready to be sent to a hospital room.

Your stay in the hospital—usually anywhere from one to ten days after surgery—will depend on the kind of surgery you have had and on your recovery rate.

Finally, your postoperative care will include the removal of any *surgical drains,* which are tubes placed in your incisions during the operation to prevent unwanted fluids from accumulating. The drains are removed at the bedside or in the clinic after three to seven days.

Pain Management

Pain after surgery for cancers of the mouth or throat is usually not as painful as some other surgeries. Whatever pain you do experience can be controlled

One of my biggest fears about surgery for cancer of the jaw bone was what I would look like and how would I function afterwards. I was so relieved when my reconstructive surgeon explained to me exactly how I was going to be "put back together."

Dave, 52
Cancer survivor

with medications; a nurse will begin administering pain medications immediately after your surgery, giving them to you on a scheduled basis if you are too groggy to ask for them. Many times, no narcotics are needed and a combination of acetaminophen and ibuprofen will be given on a scheduled basis. Medications that reduce your postoperative pain may even be given prior to the operation.

When you are awake enough, you may be able to administer your own pain medication. You can press a button on a *patient-controlled analgesia machine (PCA)*, to deliver a dose of pain medication through your IV. The machine is set so that you won't give yourself too much. (*See* chapter 8 for a more thorough discussion of pain management.)

Potential Complications

Any surgery carries potential complications. Every patient has different levels of risk, depending on the extent of their cancer, the kind of operation it requires, and his or her underlying health.

Patients occasionally develop infections. An infection can occur at the incision site. Signs of infection at the incision site include redness, warmth, pain, and drainage from the incision.

Your nurses will observe your incision while you are in the hospital; you can watch for any signs of infection after you are home.

As a recovery room nurse, my job is to protect and comfort patients as they are waking up from surgery. They can be confused by all the noises and from the medications, so I prevent them from hurting themselves and make them as relaxed as possible.

K.L.
Recovery room nurse

Pneumonia is another type of infection that can occur after surgery. Your medical team will watch for any signs of pneumonia and begin treatment immediately if needed. After you have returned home, be sure to contact your doctor immediately if you develop difficulty breathing or have fevers or chills.

Some individuals may also fail to heal well, in which case additional surgery may be needed to reconstruct the affected area.

Possible complications that can arise during or after surgery include bleeding from the surgical site. Very rare complications (less than 1 percent) include heart attack, stroke, anesthetic reaction, or death.

Usually, the more limited the surgery, the fewer the side effects and the lower the chance of complications. Many complications disappear on their own. Most others can be treated successfully, often in the period immediately following surgery.

Reconstructive Surgery

Any cancer surgery that involves the jaw, mouth, tongue, throat, or larynx can be disfiguring and can impair speech, breathing, and eating. Many of these patients need reconstructive surgery to compensate for body parts that have been removed or damaged during the surgery. The goal of reconstruction is to restore appearance and function.

Removal of Bone or Soft Tissue

There are two general rules for mouth and throat cancers. First, if bone is surgically removed, reconstruction will be required, often with little or no rehabilitation. Almost always, the repair of the jaw, cheek, floor of the mouth, or tongue are performed at the same time as the actual surgery to remove cancer.

Second, if soft tissue is removed, then reconstruction, rehabilitation, or both may be needed, depending on whether the tissue involves muscle. Reconstructive surgery typically uses either *grafts* or *flaps* of tissue from other parts of the body to replace tissue at the site being repaired.

Grafts

A graft is a piece of tissue taken from one part of the body and moved to the part of the body that needs repair. Grafts may come from skin, muscle, fat, or bone. Because grafts are pieces of tissue that are totally removed from one part of the body, they do not have their own blood supply; the grafts rely on nutrients from the site to which they are being moved. For example, in the case of a skin graft, the site to which the skin graft is applied will have underlying blood supply that will nourish the tissue. Often, a graft will come from a thin piece of skin on the thigh. As the grafted skin draws nutrients, it becomes permanently attached to its new site and gradually grows into a healthy outer layer of skin. The thigh will heal with a thin layer of scar tissue.

Flaps

There are two types of flaps. The first type of flap refers to a section of tissue that is still attached to the body by a major artery and vein or at its base. This means the flap is attached to its own blood supply. Then, it can be stretched from its original site to cover a nearby site undergoing repair. However, a *free flap* is completely

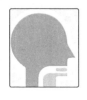

It was helpful to see a photo of a patient who had had a similar operation to mine. It gave me a sense that I could do it too.

Jessica, 70
Cancer patient

removed from the "donor" site with blood vessels attached and is then placed at the new site and the blood vessels are connected to the vessels at the new site. A flap may be taken from skin, fat, muscle, or bone.

Flaps are used more often than grafts because reconstructive surgery is usually complex enough to require an immediate supply of nutrient-rich blood. Surgical techniques using a microscope make it possible for tissue and its blood vessels to be moved from virtually any area of the body.

The kind of flap used in reconstruction depends on the kind of tissue being repaired. For example, bone flaps repair bone. One kind of bone flap uses a piece of bone from the lower leg bone to rebuild the jaw. (The removal of bone does not impair walking.) Such bone, used to rebuild the jaw bone, has its own blood supply of blood vessels, so the blood vessels in the bone are connected to blood vessels in the neck near the area of the jaw being reconstructed. Bone may also be taken from the forearm.

Commonly used skin and muscle flaps can be taken from the forearm. For example, such soft tissue flaps are used to repair the throat because the flaps are thin and pliable.

Fortunately, today, postsurgical problems of the mouth or throat can be treated successfully. If patients require functional or cosmetic surgery, this is almost always done during the main operation. The outcome might not restore 100 percent of a patient's original function or appearance, and physical therapy is usually required. But most people return to nearly normal.

Rehabilitation after Surgery

In some cases, rehabilitation, in the form of physical therapy, can resolve impairments related to surgery. For example, shoulder weakness may be caused by damage to a nerve during neck surgery to determine if cancer is present. This problem is often improved dramatically with physical therapy alone. Physical therapy also helps with other side effects such as facial and neck numbness, impairment of tongue movement, drooping of the lower lip, or, in rare cases, speech difficulties.

Radical neck dissection, which involves removal of cancer, can generate more severe side effects; they may include shoulder dysfunction, weakness, and numbness caused by damage to tissues, nerves, and veins. These problems also typically respond well to physical therapy.

The effects of removing the tongue or larynx can often be minimized with speech therapy and new techniques for eating and swallowing.

Restoring Speech

When cancer surgery significantly damages body structures that involve speech, you may need one of several aids used for speech. If your surgery required removal of your voice box, you will need to learn how to speak using one of the following three alternative methods taught by a speech therapist.

Electrolarynx. The simplest and most common of these methods uses an electrolarynx, a battery-powered device that enables an individual to form words using the mouth, lips, and tongue; the "voice" created by this device has a mechanical sound, but the method is so easy to use that most people prefer it to the others.

Tracheoesophageal puncture. Another speech method, a tracheoesophageal puncture, requires that a hole be made between the trachea and the esophagus; then, a one-way valve is inserted. This is a minor procedure, often performed on an outpatient basis. When the breathing

51

hole *(stoma)* in the lower neck is covered with a finger or valve, this forces air into the throat, causing the walls of the throat to vibrate. The sound of the vibration can then be used to form words.

Esophageal speech. Finally, a method called esophageal speech is a bit difficult to master but works well for some people. The process involves swallowing air and then belching in a controlled fashion to vibrate the throat and produce speech. This method requires no surgery or devices, and it leaves the hands free. However, for good communication, this method can be difficult to sustain a sound long enough or at a great enough volume.

Swallowing Therapy

Patients may need to work with a speech pathologist to improve swallowing after surgery, especially if part of the voice box was removed. A speech pathologist will assess the difficulty in swallowing with a modified barium swallow test. This X-ray test shows food and fluid movement during a swallow, and the various stages of swallowing may be observed. After the difficulty is pinpointed, therapies are aimed at improving the problem.

Dental Prosthesis

When a portion of the upper jaw bone is removed, it causes the cheek and lip to lose shape. In these cases, a prosthetic device, called an *obturator,* may be required. The device fits into the mouth much like a denture and fills space resulting from bone removal. The device helps restore appearance and also aids in speaking, chewing, and swallowing.

If you've had teeth removed, your surgeon may recommend dental implants. They are a special type of denture—single teeth are permanently screwed into the jaw bone.

5

RADIATION THERAPY

Almost two-thirds of people with mouth or throat cancer will receive radiation therapy. Whether radiation should be part of the treatment strategy depends on the stage of a cancer and the treatment goals. For example, if at the time of surgery the cancer is found in lymph nodes or has spread beyond the lymph nodes, radiation may improve the chance of killing any residual cancer cells.

Radiation therapy is also used in combination with chemotherapy, because these two treatments attack cancer cells through different mechanisms, potentially improving overall effectiveness. The decision to use radiation involves a careful weighing of the potential risks and side effects against the benefits. This balance is determined by your personal priorities and the probability that a given therapy will be successful. For example, radiation following surgery may improve the chances that the cancer never comes back, but it will do so at a cost to normal function. Ask your surgeon and radiation oncologist about the potential benefits and side effects of each therapy so you can make an informed decision. Medical decision making is further discussed in chapter 7. In some cases, radiation may cause less damage to tissues than surgery, so radiation may be the preferred treatment. A doctor who treats patients with radiation is called a *radiation oncologist.*

How Radiation Works

Radiation therapy uses high-powered energy waves—such as gamma rays, electron beams, and proton beams—to kill cancer cells. Cancer cells are faster growing than normal cells. Radiation kills fast-growing cells directly. Cells are most vulnerable when they are dividing. If they cannot divide, they will eventually die; they will have no new cells to replace them.

Normal cells are also damaged by radiation; however, they are able to repair the damage, whereas cancer cells typically cannot. Some normal cells also divide rapidly and are therefore damaged more than others. This is the case with cells that make up the skin and mucous membranes of the mouth and throat, so radiation often leads to sores in these areas. Fortunately, only the cells in the path of radiation are affected.

Consultation

If radiation therapy seems appropriate for you, you will have a consultation with a radiation oncologist. This doctor will examine you, review your medical records, and discuss with you in further detail the benefits and risks of radiation. Together, the two of you will decide whether you should proceed with this form of treatment. If you choose to do so, the next step is to determine which type of radiation to use and how long treatment should last.

Simulation

The planning phase of radiation treatment is called a *simulation*. During this time, CT scans will help doctors determine the placement of the radiation beam and the amount of radiation to be delivered. The dose of radiation will be calculated based on the size, extent, and type of cancer.

Pinpointing the tumor's location will determine the way your body is positioned during each radiation treatment. If you move out of position, normal cells could be

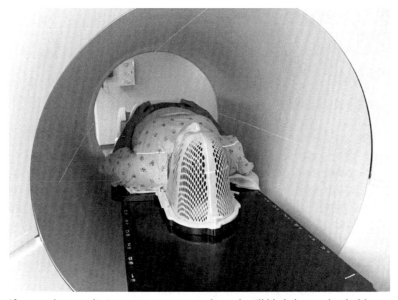

If you undergo radiation treatments, a mesh mask will likely be used to hold your head in precisely the right position during treatments.

targeted instead of cancer cells. For this reason, a technician will make a rigid mask that will go over your face, head, and neck during each treatment to hold your body in exactly the right position. If you should experience claustrophobia when such a mask is used, this can be relieved with sedatives.

The radiation oncologist and a *physicist* will work together to plan your treatment. The physicist is trained specifically in how radiation particles interact with different types of tissues and knows exactly how to direct the right dose of radiation. These doctors work together to deliver maximum radiation with minimum side effects. The plan may change during the course of your treatment if side effects become severe.

Dental Oncology Evaluation

A *dental oncologist* will evaluate you and determine whether you should have preventive dental work or extractions prior to radiation. Such an evaluation is essential. Prevention of dental problems is important to long-term care. In particular, radiation of the head or neck raises dental concerns. Radiation reduces the amount of saliva produced, changes its consistency, and reduces the blood supply to the jaw bone. These conditions promote tooth decay and brittleness.

In some situations, healthy parts of the body are protected against the effects of radiation with shields made of a lead covered with acrylic. A shield made by a dental oncologist may be used to protect key areas from radiation—especially the parotid glands, a pair of large salivary glands, one situated just in front of each ear. Protecting these glands allows the salivary glands to function more normally and to continue protecting the teeth.

Types of Radiation

Two basic types of radiation techniques are used—external and internal. External methods aim a beam of radiation at a specific body part, while internal methods involve implanting the source of radiation inside the body.

External Beam Radiation

The type of radiation most commonly used against cancers of the mouth and throat is *external beam radiation*. Radioactive beams are directed toward the body with a machine, called a *linear accelerator.* Treatments are usually given once and sometimes twice a day, five days a week for six or seven weeks. Each session takes place in a specially equipped room where you lie on a table and are moved into position by a technologist. You will wear a mask that was made for you at the start of your treatment; the mask ensures that your head remains still so that the radiation beam will be delivered precisely to the right area. After the mask is placed on your face, it will be fastened to the table to make sure you don't move your head during a treatment. Each session can last up to

I had radiation to treat cancer of the tongue. I am thankful that I am able to communicate and enjoy a great relationship with my daughters and their families. That's enough for me.

Jim, 58
Cancer survivor

ten or twenty minutes, even though the actual radiation dose is delivered painlessly in just a few seconds. The extra time is often necessary to position patients correctly on the table.

The most commonly used form of external beam therapy is *intensity-modulated radiation therapy;* it allows radiation doses to be regulated precisely for the areas being treated. The treatment is tailored to give the maximum dose of radiation to areas where a tumor is present. Lower doses are used in places that the radiation oncologist feels are unlikely to harbor any cancer. These lower doses protect normal tissues against radiation damage. Different radiation forms may also be used in some cases. For example, proton and carbon beam therapy use a heavy particle that has a better ability to be highly focused. This might lead to less toxicity to normal tissue, but the long-term results are not as well studied.

Internal Radiation Therapy

Occasionally, internal radiation, which is called *brachytherapy,* is used in mouth or throat cancers. This form of radiation is used when a high dose of radiation is required. Brachytherapy involves the implanting of radioactive "seeds" directly into the body as close to the tumor as possible. For example, when a tumor is in the base of the tongue, the seeds are implanted in the base of the tongue; the seeds can give the highest dose of radiation with the least amount of damage to surrounding normal tissue.

Brachytherapy is used most often in cases where some cancer is still present in a single location after surgery or external radiation. Brachytherapy can be either temporary or permanent.

Temporary brachytherapy. For temporary brachytherapy, a hollow tube is inserted into the treatment site, often at the time of the original cancer surgery (if the surgeon feels cancer is still present). One to five days later, the tube is loaded with radiation seeds. If extensive surgery was performed, you will need some time to heal before the seeds are placed. If not much healing time is required, the seeds can be loaded soon after surgery. The seeds are highly radioactive and so must be loaded in a hospital room that is equipped with lead shields.

This procedure is painless. After the radiation seeds have delivered the appropriate radiation dose, generally in forty-eight to seventy-two hours, the tube and seeds are removed. This removal is typically done in the patient's hospital room. While the tube is in place, however, it can transmit radiation outside the body, so contact with others is limited during this kind of treatment.

Permanent brachytherapy. This permanent form of internal therapy involves the surgical placement of radioactive seeds that remain in the body. The seeds gradually emit less and less radiation over weeks or months. This procedure may also be performed at the time of cancer surgery. It is usually performed only when the surgeon has not been able to remove all the cancer. The implanted seeds do not produce as much radiation as those used in temporary brachytherapy, so contact with other people is permitted.

Side Effects of Radiation

The side effects of radiation differ in their nature and severity for each person. Short-term side effects are those that last from weeks to months after radiation therapy has ended. Long-term side effects last longer; they might not show up for months or years, but are often permanent. Different side effects are associated with different cancer sites.

Short-Term Side Effects

Dry Mouth
Radiation damages the salivary glands that produce thin, watery saliva. The result is both less saliva and saliva that is thick and stringy; this can making swallowing difficult. Although this side effect might be temporary, it is usually permanent. If you experience this side effect, drink lots of water, and also ask about salivary substitutes. Toothpastes are available that can soothe and moisten the mouth; also, your doctor may prescribe medications that may offer some improvement. Some drugs such as antihistamines may make the dryness worse. Ask your doctor whether any of your routine medications may contribute to dry mouth. Avoid sugared or caffeinated drinks.

As for other treatments, acupuncture has been shown to help some patients improve their salivary gland function. Also, a cool mist humidifier at night may help reduce the severity of dry mouth. Special diets might be needed that don't require as much saliva to swallow. A dietician can be very helpful in selecting foods for you that might make swallowing easier.

Mucositis and Mouth Sores
An inflammation of the lining of the mouth and throat, called *mucositis,* is caused by radiation; this inflammation can occur ten to fourteen days after radiation therapy begins. If it becomes very painful, radiation may be delayed for a few days until it subsides. In the meantime, your physician may prescribe a prescription pain medication that is applied topically; he or she may also prescribe prescription mouth rinses that may help. Note

that commercial mouthwashes contain alcohol and can irritate the mouth and throat.

Sometimes radiation can lead to yeast infections in the mouth, which produce painful white sores that require antifungal medications. Other sores may occur in the mouth and throat that are similar to mucositis but are caused by a virus. These, too, can be quite painful and will require pain medicine or antiviral medication. Avoid spicy or rough-textured foods as well as tobacco, alcohol, and extremes of hot and cold food.

Difficulty Swallowing and Loss of Taste

Not only does radiation cause mouth sores and dryness that may make eating and swallowing difficult, but it also affects the taste buds so that food may lose some of its appeal. Such factors can interfere with your nutrition. Those who experience trouble eating may need to receive food through a nasogastric tube or a tube into the stomach.

You can usually avoid feeding tubes by drinking plenty of fluids to ease mouth dryness and by drinking liquid dietary supplements; these drinks provide needed calories, proteins, and vitamins. Pureed and soft foods are also usually easy to tolerate, and dips or sauces can enhance flavors. Avoid dietetic and low-fat foods; weight loss is a significant problem during and immediately after radiation treatments, so this is not the time to be use "diet" foods.

Because difficulty swallowing is often the most troublesome side effect of radiation, rehabilitation is frequently recommended. In rehab, the patient works with a speech pathologist who makes evaluations and recommendations for improving swallowing abilities both during and after completion of radiation. Patients who undergo chemotherapy along with radiation often have more swallowing difficulty than those having radiation only.

Dental Problems

Radiation reduces the production and quality of saliva, which helps clean teeth and keep them free of bacteria. As a result, saliva's cavity-fighting capability is often diminished. Even if you have shields to protect your salivary glands, you will need to see your dentist regularly to avoid or treat long-term dental problems such as decay, gum disease, and tooth fractures. In addition, a dental oncologist will probably recommend routine fluoride treatments to strengthen teeth and to prevent cavities.

Middle-Ear Fluid and Hearing Loss

When radiation is delivered to the sinus areas, swelling that results can cause fluid to accumulate in the ear and can produce associated hearing loss. This condition is reversible. Ear fluid often disappears on its own, although this can take months. Decongestants sometimes speed the process; otherwise, tubes may be placed in the ear to prevent fluid from accumulating. Tube placement is a simple surgical procedure, performed under local anesthesia. Only in uncommon cases does radiation cause permanent nerve injury, resulting in permanent hearing loss. However, when chemotherapy is given with radiation there is an increased chance of permanent hearing loss in approximately 40 percent of patients.

Eye Problems

Radiation to the sinuses can also damage the eyes, causing cataracts, pain in the eyeballs, or even blindness; however, blindness is very uncommon. If cataracts form, they can be removed by an ophthalmologist. It is very uncommon for the eyeball to receive extensive radiation, but if it does, blindness may occur, and removal of the eyeball may be necessary.

Skin Changes

Radiation can cause skin reactions, similar to sunburns. If radiation makes your skin red, dry, and irritated, wash only with gentle soap and lukewarm water. Check with your radiation therapist about using lotions or other skin products. Avoid sun exposure.

Fatigue

During the course of your radiation therapy, your body will be working to kill cancer cells and to heal from the effects of treatments. Fatigue is a natural side effect of this process, though in most cases the fatigue gradually improves after treatment has ended. In the meantime, you will need much more rest and sleep than usual, and your ability to function well at work or at home may be limited. If you discuss this likelihood with your employer and your family in advance, they will know what to expect.

Long-Term Side Effects

Bone and Tissue Injury

Radiation injuries to soft tissue, small blood vessels, and bone can diminish the blood supply to the damaged sites and ultimately lead to permanent tissue loss. Tissue injury or tissue loss, called *soft tissue necrosis,* is usually seen in areas that have received high doses of radiation. Tissue damage will usually heal on its own but can take several months. Occasionally, flaps of tissue may be needed to replace lost tissue.

Loss of bone tissue is called *osteoradionecrosis.* Radiation treatment for mouth or throat cancers can cause such bone loss in the jaw bone or other parts of the skull. Factors that cause additional risk are poor oral hygiene, dental extractions after radiation, and ongoing alcohol or tobacco abuse. One of the most likely effects of bone loss is pain, caused by lack of blood flow, infection, and inflammation; these are effects of radiation and exposed bone.

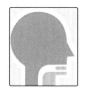

During my radiation treatments, a face mask was secured to the radiation table and it held my body still. I felt helpless but it only took a few minutes.

Pat, 72
Cancer survivor

Sometimes the effects of radiation progress to complete loss of the jaw, which requires extensive reconstructive surgery. It's not known why some patients experience continuing loss of jaw bone; however, teeth extractions appear to cause bone loss. If you need to have any teeth pulled, it is important that you tell your dentist you have had radiation to the jaw.

Treatment of such bone damage includes: removal of dead bone, improving oral hygiene, and possibly the use of *hyperbaric oxygen (HBO)*—oxygen delivered to the entire body under high pressure. This treatment helps the body form new blood vessels. This process increases the oxygen and nutrients delivered to bone, allowing the bone to heal much faster. However, HBO cannot restore dead bone structures.

Any dead bone must be removed either before HBO begins or during the course of treatment. Removal of dead bone is sometimes done in a doctor's office with local anesthetic, but sometimes it requires a surgery with general anesthesia. The type of surgery needed depends on the amount of bone to be removed and the depth of the dead bone in the jaw.

HBO treatments are given daily. Each one lasts about ninety minutes; a patient is placed in a small tank but is able to see out. This tank is pressurized and can make you feel like you dived thirty-two to forty-five feet under water. Most people tolerate the treatments well, but if you have claustrophobia you can ask your doctor for medication to lessen the symptoms. Some people also need ear tubes if they experience significant ear pressure and pain during the therapy.

Chronic Skin Changes

Radiation may result in scarring of the skin and its underlying structures. Such a side effect gradually turns soft skin into hard and "woody" skin; sometimes this side effect is permanent. It is more likely to happen if you have previously undergone surgery or chemotherapy. It is hard to predict who will have these changes in their skin. Good skin care, moisturizers, and sun avoidance can minimize these side effects.

Decreased Thyroid Function

Radiation can permanently injure the thyroid gland, preventing or limiting its production of the thyroid hormone. This hormone regulates the function of every organ in your body. If production of this hormone is impaired, all normal body functions slow down.

It's important to have your thyroid function checked six to twelve months after your treatment ends. Fortunately, thyroid hormone can easily be replaced with medication taken once a day.

Chronic Swelling

Swelling of the neck—especially under the chin—may persist after radiation therapy. This is known as *lymphedema*. Lymphedema is swelling caused by fluid buildup that may occur after radiation and/or surgical removal of lymph nodes. Usually, neck swelling resolves in six months to a year; however, it can last for years. Such swelling is often worse in the mornings. Many patients fear that this swelling might represent a recurrence of cancer, since it often doesn't show up until several months after radiation therapy, and it may feel like a lump under the chin.

Lymphedema specialists may work with you to decrease the swelling and improve recovery. These specialists use massage in an effort to lessen fluid buildup. Also, keeping your head elevated when you sleep may be helpful. Still, time is the best remedy, and this kind of swelling usually resolves on its own.

Swelling of the larynx can affect the quality of your voice as well as create difficulty breathing. In rare instances, a tracheostomy tube (inserted in the windpipe) is necessary until the swelling resolves. Swelling in this area often worsens right after radiation has ended, then it usually begins to resolve in four to eight weeks. Rarely, the swelling lasts for years or is permanent.

Swelling of the tongue, pharyngeal walls, palate, or uvula can impede speech and swallowing. Again, this may require a tracheostomy or feeding tube until the swelling resolves, usually in a couple of months.

Decreased Jaw Opening

Radiation-induced scars in the jaw joint and surrounding tissues create a condition called *trismus,* an inability to open the mouth all the way. Stretching exercises can relieve this condition, and if the exercises are started early, they can even prevent the condition. Your dental oncologist will direct you in the proper mouth-opening exercises.

Secondary Cancer Formation

There is a low risk of radiation causing a new cancer many years later at the site that received radiation treatment. If this should occur, the cancer will be surgically removed.

6

CHEMOTHERAPY, TARGETED THERAPY, AND IMMUNOTHERAPY

The word chemotherapy may raise fear and uncertainty in your mind—no doubt because in the past, its benefits have often come at the cost of serious side effects. Fortunately, newer types of chemotherapy drugs have been proven to be increasingly successful in battling cancer, with reduced overall side effects. In addition, medications given with chemotherapy to prevent and treat side effects, especially for nausea and vomiting, also have improved.

Nowadays, the term *chemotherapy* encompasses not only traditional chemotherapy, but also more recent treatments—*targeted therapy* and *immunotherapy*. All of these treatments can be thought of as part of a broad category of "systemic" therapy, meaning whole-body treatment, as opposed to surgery and radiation therapy, which are both "localized" treatments.

How Chemotherapy Works

Like radiation therapy, traditional chemotherapy drugs work against cells that are reproducing quickly. As mentioned earlier, cancer cells are rapidly growing cells. Different drugs used in chemotherapy work against these cells in different ways. Most traditional chemotherapy drugs work by interfering with some portion of a cell's division process. And, when a combination of drugs is used, the advantages of each drug can be maximized, creating better results than one drug alone.

Because traditional chemotherapy also affects rapidly dividing normal cells, this leads to side effects in healthy cells. For example, quickly growing cells are found in the hair, in the lining of the mouth, and in the blood. As a result, side effects may include hair loss, mouth sores, or low white blood cell levels. Later in this chapter, side effects of chemotherapy are discussed in detail, along with strategies to manage them.

Are You a Candidate for Chemotherapy?

Whether you will need chemotherapy depends on the specific type of cancer you have, how advanced it is, and the treatment goal. Chemotherapy alone can be curative in some other kinds of cancer, but to be part of a curative treatment for patients with mouth or throat cancer, it must be used in combination with surgery or radiation therapy.

If you do need chemotherapy as part of your treatment plan, you and your doctor will have a detailed discussion. He or she will talk to you about the benefits and risks of the specific chemotherapy treatments you would be receiving. A physician who specializes in chemotherapy treatment is called a *medical oncologist.*

Receiving Chemotherapy

To help you decide if you will undergo chemotherapy, you will meet with a medical oncologist. During an initial consultation, the oncologist will examine you, review your medical records, and recommend which drugs to use, how to deliver them, and for how long a time. He or she will review with you the risks and benefits of treatment.

Delivery of Treatment

Most chemotherapy drugs are infused through an IV line into a small vein, usually in the arm or hand. Some drugs are too harsh for these small veins, however. In this case, or if you need multiple treatments, several other options are available. A central venous catheter or "port" can be inserted surgically into a larger vein and left in place until your course of therapy is complete. In some cases, the drugs are taken by mouth.

Chemotherapy can be administered in the hospital, a clinic, a doctor's office, or even in the home. It is usually done on an outpatient basis, but this depends on the drugs used and how well you tolerate them.

Duration and Frequency of Treatment

Your chemotherapy treatments could be given daily, weekly, or monthly for a period up to several months. The overall plan depends on your cancer, your condition, and your tolerance for the drugs. For example, your treatment will take longer if you need extra time between sessions to recuperate from the effects of the drugs.

You might even need a break—several days or weeks off from chemotherapy—if your side effects are severe or your blood counts are low. The actual delivery of chemotherapy is not painful, though the sessions can last up to several hours. It feels like any other IV fluids going into the vein.

Chemotherapy Side Effects

Chemotherapy causes side effects when normal cells are damaged. You may experience some, all, or none of the side effects discussed below. The side effects may be mild or severe. Most will gradually disappear after chemotherapy treatment is completed, though some can cause permanent damage. Depending on the drugs used and their dosages, the effects usually intensify if chemotherapy is coupled with radiation.

The following is a general list of side effects seen with various chemotherapy drugs, and is derived from materials from the National Institutes of Health. If you need chemotherapy as part of your treatment, your medi-

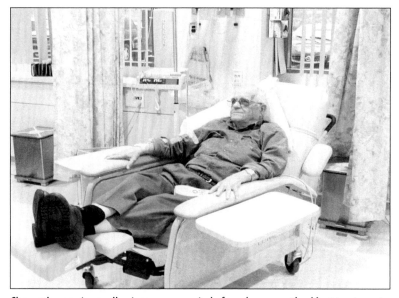

Chemotherapy is usually given over a period of weeks or months. Most treatments, called *infusions,* are giving intravenously at at hospital or clinic.

cal oncologist will have a detailed discussion with you regarding the expected and potential side effects of your specific chemotherapy treatment plan, which may differ significantly from this general list. In particular, immuno-therapy and targeted therapies generally have very different side effects compared to traditional chemotherapies. Targeted therapy and immunotherapy and their side effects are discussed at the end of this chapter.

Hair Loss

Chemotherapy very commonly causes hair from all parts of the body to thin, fall out gradually, or come out in large clumps. In most cases, the hair grows back after chemotherapy, though sometimes the color or texture of the new hair is different. To take care of your hair and scalp during chemotherapy, follow these recommendations:

- Use mild shampoos.
- Use a soft hairbrush.
- Set your hair dryer on low.
- Don't use brush rollers or heated rollers to set your hair.
- Don't use hair color or permanents.
- Cut your hair short, so it will look fuller.
- Cover your scalp when you are in the sun.

If your hair thins or falls out, you might want to wear a wig, scarf, hat, or other head covering. Some cancer organizations specialize in helping cancer patients with headdresses or makeup. If you plan to wear a wig, it is a good idea to purchase one before your treatments begin so you can match your hair color and texture.

Nausea and Vomiting

Chemotherapy drugs can affect the stomach lining or the area of the brain that controls vomiting. Fortunately, both nausea and vomiting are better controlled than ever by new medications. Traditional chemotherapy is given in conjunction with what are called "pre-medications" to try to prevent or treat nausea and vomiting. Just prior to chemotherapy, sometimes three or four medications are given all together that each work to try to prevent nausea in completely different ways. Drugs can work differently for different people, so don't give up if one or two do not work for you; your medical oncologist and you will work together to find the combination of medications that works best. The following techniques can also help:

- Do eat modest regular meals on the days of your chemotherapy appointments. Don't go on an empty stomach.
- Avoid large meals. Instead, eat several small meals during the day.
- Eat and drink slowly. Chew your food well.

- Wear loose-fitting clothes.
- Avoid strong odors.
- Suck on ice chips, mints, or tart candies, unless you have mouth sores.
- Use deep breathing or other relaxation methods when you feel nauseated.

Diarrhea

Chemotherapy drugs can affect the lining of the large intestine, producing loose or watery stools. If diarrhea lasts more than twenty-four hours or is accompanied by abdominal pain or cramping, tell your doctor. If your diarrhea persists, your doctor may prescribe medications or order intravenous fluids to guard against dehydration. You can prevent diarrhea, or ease it, in the following ways:

- Eat smaller amounts of food more often.
- Avoid foods that are high in fiber, such as raw fruits and vegetables, whole grains, beans, seeds, and nuts.
- Avoid coffee, tea, alcohol, sugar, spicy foods, and fried foods.
- Drink plenty of fluids.

Also, consult your doctor before taking any over-the-counter medications.

Decreased Blood Counts

Chemotherapy can reduce your bone marrow's ability to make red blood cells, white blood cells, and platelets. Blood counts of each of these types of cells are likely to drop seven to fourteen days after a chemotherapy treatment. Each kind of blood cell has an important function, so when their levels drop, their function is compromised and an associated risk arises.

Anemia. Red blood cells carry oxygen throughout the body. A decrease in red blood cell production can lead to

---

Palliative Care

When a cure is not possible, chemotherapy is usually used alone, as *palliative cancer treatment.* The intent is to shrink the cancer or slow its growth and primarily to reduce symptoms caused by the cancer itself. The goal is to prolong life and improve quality of life. Potential side effects can vary greatly, depending on the drugs used.

---

anemia. Symptoms of anemia include dizziness, fatigue, and breathlessness. A healthy, well-balanced diet and iron supplements can minimize this risk. If your anemia becomes serious, you may need a blood transfusion.

Infection. White blood cells prevent infection, so when their count is low you are more susceptible to infections. There are steps you can take to reduce your risk:

- Stay away from people with colds, the flu, or other contagious diseases.
- Wash your hands often, especially after using the bathroom.
- Keep your skin clean and smooth so that bacteria cannot enter.
- Clean your rectal area thoroughly after each bowel movement. Tell your doctor if this area becomes sore or if you have hemorrhoids.
- Avoid children or adults who have recently received vaccinations.
- Clean cuts or scrapes immediately.
- Wear gloves for gardening and housecleaning.
- Avoid tasks or tools that could cause nicks or cuts.
- Use a soft toothbrush and floss gently, so your gums don't bleed.

Although infection can involve virtually any area of your body, it arises most often in the skin, gums, lungs, bowels, bladder, sinuses, and throat. Infections can be fatal when your white blood cell count is very low, so you should report any of the following symptoms to your doctor:

- Fever over 100.5 degrees F
- Chills
- Sweating
- Discomfort or burning during urination
- Severe cough or sore throat
- Unusual vaginal discharge or itching
- Redness, swelling, tenderness, or discharge, especially around a catheter, wound, incision, sore, or pimple

Do not take aspirin or acetaminophen for any of these symptoms without first checking with your doctor.

Blood Clotting Problems

Platelets—another type of cell produced by the bone marrow—are necessary to the formation of blood clots. When your skin is injured or broken, platelets clump together and form clots to stop the bleeding. A low platelet count makes you more susceptible to bleeding and bruising. With a severely low platelet count, even a minor injury can bleed persistently or cause severe bruising. You might even develop spontaneous nosebleeds or see blood in your urine or stool. These side effects can be severe. You should notify your doctor if a nosebleed does not stop after pressure has been applied for ten to fifteen minutes or if the amount of blood in your stool or urine is large. To minimize the problems associated with poor blood clotting, take the following precautions:

- Avoid aspirin and ibuprofen, which can further impair platelet function. Always check with your doctor before taking any medication.

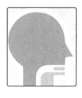

The worst part of radiation was that food did not have much taste, and when it did, it was often bad. The good news is that it does get better. Now I eat whatever I want, and it is great.

Carl, 52
Cancer survivor

- Do not drink alcohol without first checking with your doctor.
- Brush your teeth gently with a soft brush.
- Use caution in all your activities—especially in the kitchen, bathroom, or any area where minor injuries are common.
- Blow your nose gently.
- Handle scissors, knives, and tools with extra care.

If your platelet counts become dangerously low, you will probably be given a platelet transfusion. When a platelet count is 70,000 or higher, the risk of bleeding is low. When it falls below 20,000, the risk of spontaneous bleeding begins to increase but probably does not become severe until the count is 5,000 to 10,000.

A transfusion of platelets prevents dangerous bleeding when the platelet count is between 10,000 and 20,000. However in some cases, a transfusion may not be necessary unless the platelet count drops to 5,000.

Nerve Problems

Some chemotherapy drugs affect nerves; and depending on which nerves are affected, symptoms may include hearing loss, ringing in the ears, poor balance, or numbness, burning, and tingling in the hands and feet. These effects may or may not be permanent. Talk to your doctor about managing such symptoms.

If you are having difficulty with balance:

- Be careful getting in and out of the tub or shower.
- Use the handrails on stairs.
- Use a cane if necessary.
- Avoid sharp or dangerous objects, or handle them with extra care.
- Do not wear loose or slippery shoes or sandals.

In some cases, numbness goes away or becomes less severe, but not always. Most patients, even those with permanent effects of nerve damage, learn to adjust to these problems.

Mouth and Throat Sores

Chemotherapy can cause mouth dryness, irritate the tissues of the mouth and throat, or produce sores or ulcers that sometimes bleed and always carry some risk of infection. If you have sores in your mouth, ask your doctor whether medications can help. In the meantime, practice good oral hygiene:

- Try to see your dentist or dental oncologist before chemotherapy to have your teeth cleaned and any cavities filled.
- Brush and floss regularly but gently.
- Use a soft toothbrush, rinse it well, and store it in a dry place.
- Avoid commercial mouthwashes, which usually contain salt and alcohol. Ask your doctor, dentist, or nurse to recommend a mouthwash or oral care gel.

To ease the discomfort of mouth sores:

- Ask for pain medication from your doctor.
- Eat foods cold or at room temperature. (Heat can irritate sore tissues.)
- Choose soft, bland foods.
- Avoid acidic and spicy foods.

To relieve mouth dryness:
- Drink plenty of fluids.
- Moisten foods with butter or sauces.
- Suck on ice chips or hard candies.
- Use lip balm.
- Eat soft foods.

Effects on Major Organs

As a systemic therapy that travels through the whole body, chemotherapy drugs can affect virtually any part of the body—even the heart, liver, or kidneys. Routine blood tests are used to monitor liver and kidney function. If the tests indicate a problem with any organ function, this could require a reduction in your dose of chemotherapy medication or a switch to another drug.

The heart can be monitored by an *electrocardiogram (EKG),* which records the heart's electrical impulses, or an *echocardiogram,* which uses ultrasound to measure cardiac function. Sometimes a *stress test* (such as a treadmill test) is used to check on the heart's function during physical exertion. Depending on the specific chemotherapy drugs you need, these tests may or may not be needed routinely.

If you experience any chest pain, shortness of breath, or changes in the amount or characteristics of your urine, be sure to report these to your doctor.

Skin and Nail Changes

Chemotherapy can increase the skin's sensitivity to the sun, causing rashes when you are outdoors even for short periods of time, especially in the hottest times of day. Be sure to cover your skin. Wear sunscreen, hats, and long-sleeved shirts. This effect is most pronounced during the period of treatment, but it can linger for months. It is uncomfortable and annoying, even though the rashes are not dangerous. Knowing the link between sun exposure

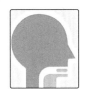

Some chemotherapy causes your hair to fall out and you may lose weight. It is scary, but believe me, you can do it. But, you can't beat this disease alone. Trust your doctors. Let your loved ones love and help you.

Denise, 42
Cancer survivor

and skin cancer, however, it is a good idea to make sun protection a way of life.

If your fingernails change to yellow or a darker color, or if they become ridged or brittle, you can use over-the-counter nail strengtheners. Wearing gloves for household chores and gardening can also help protect your nails.

Most skin changes caused by chemotherapy are temporary and fairly mild. However, more serious damage can be done if a drug leaks out of a vein during a treatment session. This can injure the skin and surrounding tissue. Be sure to tell your doctor or technician immediately if you feel pain or burning as the drugs are being given. Also inform your doctor if you develop severe itching or rashes, if you begin wheezing, or if you have trouble breathing. These can all be signs of an allergic reaction, which is a rare but known potential side effect of certain chemotherapy drugs.

Sexual and Reproductive Changes

Chemotherapy can affect the sexual organs, sexual function, and fertility in both men and women. Some people note an increased desire for intimacy; others find it difficult to respond sexually because of the physical and emotional stress of treatment. Good and supportive communication with your partner is most important at this time—especially if he or she is worried that intimate contact might harm you.

Infertility associated with chemotherapy can be temporary or permanent. Some men consider banking sperm before they begin their treatments. Some women who are still of childbearing age may wish to speak with their oncologist about using a chemotherapy drug that decreases the chances of infertility.

In women, reduced hormone production can produce menopause-like symptoms, including irregular menstrual periods, hot flashes, itching, burning, and vaginal dryness. Water-soluble vaginal lubricants can help, and wearing "breathable" cotton underwear can reduce the risk of infection caused by vaginal dryness.

Both men and women of all ages who are sexually active should use birth control during the course of chemotherapy treatments and for at least three months after completion because the drugs can be harmful to a fetus. If you think you might want a child in the future, you may wish to see a reproductive specialist before you start chemotherapy.

Targeted Therapy

Targeted therapy refers to systemic medications that have been tailored to attack an individual's cancer cells in a specific way that is different from the way traditional chemotherapies work. Targeted therapy has been used in the treatment of head and neck cancers since the mid-2000s.

How Targeted Therapy Works

There are different kinds of targeted therapy drugs that work in a variety of ways. Some targeted therapies inactivate proteins on the surface of cancer cells. Some targeted therapies work against cancer cells by inactivating certain proteins inside the cancer cell that are responsible for a cancer cell's ability to grow and spread. Other targeted therapies work by inactivating proteins within cancer cells that otherwise would allow mutated DNA instructions to be carried out. Still other targeted therapies don't work on the cancer cell itself, rather they work on the tissues necessary for the cancer's survival. For example, some targeted therapies work against the formation of the new blood vessels that feed a tumor.

Are You a Candidate for Targeted Therapy?

To determine if you are a candidate for targeted therapy, your physician may need to order specific tests on your cancer cells to determine if the molecular target needed for a particular drug to work is present. Your physician may need to order tests on tissue samples from biopsies of your tumor, or may order blood tests. The term *liquid biopsy* is sometimes used to refer to tests on blood and possibly other bodily fluids such as urine that may help your doctor determine the best treatment for your situation.

Receiving Targeted Therapy

Targeted therapy includes a group of medicines that work in very different ways and are also given in very different ways. Your physician will discuss with you the details of how you would receive targeted therapy if it is part of your treatment plan. Some treatments are delivered intravenously (IV) and others are taken by mouth. The schedules for targeted therapy vary. Some are given once weekly by IV. Others are given once monthly by IV or once daily by mouth.

The duration of treatment also varies, depending on your treatment goals. Some regimens are given for a fixed amount of time, and some are given on an ongoing basis as long as you and your oncologist consider it beneficial.

Side Effects of Targeted Therapy

Because targeted therapy drugs focus on attacking cancer cells, fewer healthy cells are affected compared with traditional chemotherapy. Therefore, patients treated with targeted therapy generally experience milder and different side effects. Nausea, vomiting, and hair loss are often not seen at all with some targeted therapy drugs.

Still, some of the common side effects of targeted therapies include an acne-like rash, dry skin, fatigue, diarrhea, and low magnesium or potassium blood levels. Rare but potentially severe side effects include allergic reaction during the IV infusion and severe skin reactions. It is important to know, though, that even in the category of targeted therapy, individual drugs can work entirely differently from others, resulting in very different side effects.

Immunotherapy

The immune system is a complex network that protects us from infections, foreign cells, and abnormal cells such as cancer cells. The most significant recent advance in chemotherapy treatment for head and neck cancers is the FDA approval in 2017 of a new group of drugs called *PD-1 immune checkpoint inhibitors.* These drugs work by increasing the ability of the body's own immune cells to identify and attack cancer cells.

At present, the PD-1 immune checkpoint inhibitors for the treatment of mouth and throat cancers have been shown to be effective only to improve cancer control for patients with incurable disease; however, research continues to determine whether these drugs can work in conjunction with radiation therapy or surgery to increase the chance for cure.

How Immunotherapy Works

One key part of the immune system is a particular type of white blood cell called a *T-cell;* this cell identifies and attacks cancer cells while leaving normal healthy cells alone.

When the T-cell encounters another cell, there are multiple "checkpoint" molecules that tell the T-cell whether to attack or leave the cell alone. One of the major checkpoint inhibitor systems, the *PD-1 (programmed cell death protein-1)* system, works as an "off-switch" to tell the T-cell to ignore normal cells but to attack cancer cells. However, cancer cells can take advantage of the PD-1 system—the cells can escape being attacked by the body's T-cells by being able to signal through the PD-1 system that they are normal cells and should be left alone. New immunotherapies block the PD-1 system, which allows T-cells to recognize the cell as an abnormal cell so the T-cell can attack.

Receiving Immunotherapy

The current FDA-approved targeted immunotherapy agents are given intravenously, once every three weeks or once every four weeks, depending on the specific drug being given.

Side Effects of Immunotherapy

Side effects of PD-1 inhibitor treatment are generally mild for the majority of patients. In fact, the majority of patients have no side effects. Still, rare but potentially severe side effects are possible as a result of immune "over-activation." This means the body's immune system may become too active in the lungs, colon, skin, liver, kidneys, and endocrine glands; this can cause side effects such as shortness of breath, diarrhea, rash, elevation in liver or kidney blood tests, or low thyroid function. If these side effects should occur, they can almost always be treated effectively by your physician, and immunotherapy can continue.

The Importance of Support

Undergoing any of the therapies, especially chemotherapy, described in this chapter may be difficult at times for both you and your family. The length of treatment can seem long and the side effects distressing. Do not hesitate to seek the support you need from your doctors, nurses, family, friends, a counselor, or support group. Above all, ask questions of your medical team so that you can be informed and play an active role in your treatment.

7

TREATING CANCER BY STAGE

The process of *staging* a cancer involves determining the extent of a cancer's growth. Is the cancer at an early stage? Or has is spread beyond the site of origin? Knowing the stage of a cancer is important because it is one factor that helps doctors determine the best treatment.

To determine the stage of cancer, doctors need to know:

- The size of the tumor
- The extent of tumor growth
- Whether lymph nodes near the tumor are involved and their size and location
- Whether the cancer has spread to other organs

There are two types of staging: clinical and pathological. *Clinical staging* is based on a physical examination and diagnostic tests, including X-rays, scans—such as computerized tomography (CT) and magnetic resonance imaging (MRI), and biopsies—prior to any treatment. A clinical stage is determined for every patient.

Pathological staging is based on the clinical findings along with an analysis of tumor samples after surgery, if surgery has been performed. If surgery has not been performed, pathologic staging cannot be done and the staging is only based on the clinical findings such as biopsies and imaging scans.

Treatment Plan

The treatment used depends on the location and stage of the cancer being treated as well as on a patient's age and health. Many variables affect the kind of treatment you will receive for your cancer. If you wish to be informed and involved in the choices that go into your treatment, let your doctors know. Ask that all the options be reviewed with you so that you will understand the advantages and disadvantages.

From the physicians' standpoint, the relevant factors in any treatment are its effectiveness and your ability to withstand its likely side effects or complications. From your standpoint, you may wonder what emotional and psychological trade-offs are involved. These are considerations you will want to discuss with your physicians. This is a process known as *medical decision making.*

Medical Decision Making

Your doctors will study each of three factors to make a plan for you. These factors include tumor factors, treatment options available and your overall health. The tumor factors include things such as the site, stage, grade, and specific tumor type. Also, what vital structures will be affected by treatment such as the upper and lower jaw, larynx (voice box), or teeth?

Your doctors, along with your primary care doctor or specialists, will determine if you are healthy enough to undergo specific treatments. Finally, the doctors will determine if there is another type of treatment that is not available at their institution that might provide a higher cure rate or perhaps fewer complications. All of these factors are put together at a *tumor board meeting* to provide a plan that is designed to provide the highest cure rate without excessive complications.

Tumor Board Meetings

As part of the team approach, cancer specialists in most major cancer centers have a weekly conference during which new patients' cases are presented to a board of specialists for their recommendations. The appropriate images, either photographic, radiographic, or ultrasound, are shown by a radiologist. Also, a microscopic image of the cancer is shown to the group by a pathologist, and the treating physician presents information about the patient and the cancer's stage. The group has an in-depth discussion about the best options for each patient. These options are then presented to the patient for shared medical decision making and a final plan is developed.

Personal Choices

The next step in medical decision making is the crucial discussion about what you want. Only you and your family can make known your wishes. Most patients want the treatment that will give them the highest chance of being cured and will agree with the plan created in the tumor board meeting. However, some people who learn their chances of a cure are only 10 to 15 percent may consider it more important to them to avoid certain side effects than to get the highest cure rate.

Examples of this might be avoiding the dry mouth, reduced sense of taste, fatigue, and difficulty swallowing that often occurs after radiation. Each person is unique, and therefore each decision is unique. Make sure you express your wishes to your doctors. You want them to be able to consider the pros and cons of each step in the decision making process; they want you to understand the relative benefits and downsides to each treatment approach.

Multimodality Therapy

A combination of treatments—surgery, radiation, and chemotherapy—have long been used in the treatment of

When they told me that I had to have chemotherapy and then radiation, I did not think I could do it. The love of my family pulled me through. I remembered my doctor telling me to set some goals. My goal was to see my son play football as a senior, and I did!

David, 45
Cancer survivor

cancer, but, increasingly, they are being administered in new and varying combinations, dosages, and sequences. This fine-tuned approach is called *multimodality therapy.* It refers to using more than one mode of treatment. A team of specialists work together, from the beginning of a patient's diagnosis; they consult, strategize, and deliver the most promising combination of up-to-date treatments. This meeting is known as a *multidisciplinary tumor board.* As a result, you may not need to visit a series of doctors. Instead, with the multimodality approach, you will likely be sent directly to one specialist who will oversee your treatment.

Treatment Strategies

The following sections describe in a general way the circumstances and conditions under which single therapies and multimodal therapies might be used to treat various stages of cancer. These discussions also cover some of the benefits and difficulties associated with the different forms of treatment. The chart on page 87 shows the treatment options for various stages of cancers of the mouth and throat. It is important to remember that stage is only one of many factors that go into treatment recommendations.

Surgery for Early- and Late-Stage Cancer

Nearly every kind of squamous cell mouth or throat cancer can be treated with surgery alone if it is caught and

Treatment by Stage for Head and Neck Cancer

	Surgery alone	Radiation alone	Surgery followed by radiation	Chemotherapy* with surgery, radiation, or both
Mouth				
Lip	I ,II, III	I ,II, III	III, IV	III, IV
Tongue	I ,II, III	I ,II, III	II, III, IV	III, IV
Cheek mucosa	I ,II, III	I ,II, III	II, III, IV	III, IV
Floor of mouth	I ,II, III	I ,II, III	II, IV	III, IV
Lower gum	I ,II, III	I ,II, III	III, IV	IV
Upper gum	I ,II, III	I ,II, III	II, III, IV	III, IV
Throat				
Larynx				
Supraglottis	I ,II, III	I ,II, III	II, IV	III, IV
Glottis	I ,II, III	I ,II, III	III, IV	III, IV
Subglottis	I, II	I ,II, III	III, IV	III, IV
Hypopharynx	I, II	I, II	II, III, IV	II, III, IV
Oropharynx	I ,II, III	I ,II, III	III, IV	III, IV
Nasopharynx		I, II		III, IV
Paranasal Sinuses				
Maxillary	I, II	I, II	I, II	III, IV
Ethmoid	I, II	I, II	I, II	III, IV
Nasal cavity	I, II, III, IV	I, II, III, IV	I, II, III, IV	III, IV
Salivary Gland				
High-grade	I, II	I, II	I, II, III, IV	III, IV
Low-grade	I, II		II, III, IV	III, IV

*Chemotherapy is a rapidly changing field and is often considered experimental. In the case of mouth and throat cancers, it is usually done as part of a clinical trial.

treated in the early stages, before it has grown very large or has spread beyond its original site. In most stage I and stage II cancers, surgery can often remove all cancerous tissue and cure the disease. An exception to this general rule are cancers with an HPV origin. Another exception is cancer of the nasopharynx, which is the upper part of the cavity behind the nose and mouth, and is difficult to surgically remove and is better treated with radiation in the early stages.

Because the cure rates are very high for human papillomavirus (HPV)–associated cancers of the oropharynx (tonsils and base of tongue), the treatments for these cancers are being carefully studied to determine the best treatment with the fewest long-term side effects. At this time, surgery, oftentimes followed by lower-dose radiation and possibly chemotherapy, may be recommended for stage I cancers; in other medical centers, higher-dose radiation with or without chemotherapy is used.

A few later-stage cancers—those that are small or have spread to only one lymph node in the neck (stages III and IV)—can also be treated with surgery alone. For example, in a stage III cancer on the floor of the mouth or in the nasal cavity, surgery might succeed in removing both the original cancer and any lymph nodes to which it has spread. Occasionally, a stage IV cancer of the larynx may be treated with surgery alone, if it is fairly large but has invaded no lymph nodes at all or only one lymph node.

In addition, as the chart shows stage IV cancer of the nasal cavity can be treated with only surgery. These tumors are designated stage IV if they go through the inside of the nose to the outside, a relatively short distance and therefore easier to manage surgically.

In general, cancers caught in early stages require less extensive surgery or radiation than later-stage cancers because they are usually smaller and have not spread to other structures. In the various mouth cancers, surgery

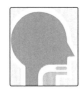

I saw so many specialists that I had trouble remembering everyone's role in my treatment. I felt out of control. It was helpful that my surgeon told me that he was the "captain of the ship" and was directing all my care.

Al, 67
Cancer patient

can mean minimal loss of the tissues of the tongue, lip, cheek, or other structures. In cancers of the larynx (voice box), surgery can be limited to procedures such as a simple removal of the cancer, a *cordectomy* (removal of a vocal cord) or, a *partial laryngectomy* (removal of some or all of the voice box).

However, when a cancer has developed close to bone, surgery may be more invasive. For example, when a mouth cancer is located near the jaw bone but does not seem to have invaded it, part of the jaw bone may still be taken out along with the cancer as a precaution against cancer recurring in the same area. In some cases, only the inner part of the jaw bone needs to be removed, making reconstruction relatively easier. The bone will be tested for cancer cells by the pathologist. Where bone is taken, reconstructive surgery is usually required. However, no further treatment may be needed for the cancer itself—only regular follow-up examinations to check for recurrences.

Radiation for Early- and Late-Stage Cancer

Stage I and II cancers of the larynx are most commonly treated with radiation therapy alone; this treatment is used when surgery is too difficult or destructive. This is often the case when large amounts of tissue would result in loss of function, or when the patient's health is fragile. External radiation is used with the intent to focus on a small area, limiting the exposure of nearby healthy tissue, and decreasing side effects. Internal radiation (brachytherapy) is usually not needed for early-stage disease.

Nearly every early-stage mouth or throat cancer can be treated with radiation alone, although surgery is preferred whenever possible. In low-grade (slow-growing) salivary gland cancers, surgery alone is more effective in almost all cases. For early cancers of the nasopharynx, radiation alone is the treatment of choice, even though it must be delivered with great care to avoid vital nearby structures such as the brain, eyes, and the nerves that supply the sensation and critical motion to the eyes.

Some stage III and even some stage IV cancers can be treated with radiation alone. This is the case if a patient cannot undergo surgery or if both the primary cancer and the sites to which it has spread are responsive to radiation. The ability of radiation to kill cancer decreases as the cancer itself advances. Sometimes, however, higher doses of radiation will succeed in treating stage III or IV cancers, especially with the addition of chemotherapy. It is more likely, however, that some combination of radiation, chemotherapy, and surgery will be required.

Combining Treatment Options

Surgery Followed by Radiation with or without Chemotherapy

Any cancer for which surgery is the first treatment option can require radiation and sometimes chemotherapy as well, either immediately after the surgery or some time later. Surgery helps determine whether additional therapy is called for because the surgery provides both a direct examination at the tumor and a pathological analysis of it. Therapy that follows another form of treatment is known as *adjuvant therapy*.

Radiation therapy is generally recommended after surgery in the following instances:

- When the tumor is large (T4)
- When cancer is deeply invasive (especially into blood vessels or nerves)

- When more than one lymph node is cancerous
- When the cancer is high-grade (fast-growing)—a designation used mainly for sarcomas and salivary gland cancers

Radiation with chemotherapy is usually recommended in these cases:

- When a tissue margin has cancer cells
- When the cancer cannot be removed completely
- When a single lymph node shows cancer extending outside the capsule of the node

In each of these situations listed, postsurgical radiation with or without chemotherapy improves the odds, but does not guarantee that cancer will not recur. A pathologist's analysis of tissue removed during surgery will help clarify the prognosis. Complications from therapy also need to be considered in the medical decision making.

Although tumors tend to be larger at later stages, even small ones can be difficult to remove completely. Thus, radiation might be required to kill residual cancer cells at any stage of the disease. Again, treatment depends on the cancer's primary site. Cancers of the paranasal sinuses (behind the nasal cavity) can require both surgery and radiation even in the earlier stages; most other cancers of the mouth and throat tend to require this combination only at stage III or IV.

Radiation Followed by Surgery

Surgery may be called for when radiation alone has failed to kill all the cancer. This happens much less often than the reverse (surgery first, radiation after) because no pathological analysis is available to indicate who will benefit from surgery after radiation. In general, surgery is used if either the primary site or the lymph nodes remain abnormal after radiation treatments have been completed, or if the cancer recurs months or years later. But the side effects of radiation can weaken patients, making them less likely candidates for surgery.

Chemotherapy with Radiation

When surgery and radiation seem unlikely to eliminate cancer, the next consideration involves chemotherapy in combination with radiation. This approach may be recommended with stage III and stage IV cancers, and occasionally in stage II cancers of the hypopharynx, a particularly aggressive disease. The hypopharynx is toward the back of the throat at the entrance into the esophagus, which carries food to the stomach. It is important to realize that chemotherapy alone does not cure cancers of the mouth and throat and that it must be used in combination with radiation.

Alternative and Complementary Therapies

Some cancer patients decide to explore therapies regarded as being outside mainstream medical practice in Western nations. These therapies may have benefits, but they have not undergone the same controlled, rigorous testing as standard treatments. Such alternative therapies may improve the quality of life of cancer patients; however, what has not been proven is that these alternative treatments increase the survival rate.

Therapies such as massage, relaxation, biofeedback, acupuncture, and meditation may be beneficial and have little potential to do harm. However, herbs are another matter. Many herbs contain powerful substances, none of which are regulated by the Food and Drug Administration. Accordingly, use herbs cautiously and only after discussing the matter with your physician.

Changes in Cancer Treatment

The treatment strategies covered in this chapter are subject to change all the time, as new and more sophisticated therapies and combinations become available through research and testing. With each new improvement, chances for a full recovery from cancer and its side effects also improve.

As you and your doctors examine the strategies available to you, the process will probably lead you to one of the options discussed in this chapter. Or, it could lead you to cutting-edge treatments still being tested.

8

Pain Management

Understandably, pain is one of the things that cancer patients fear the most. Fortunately, this fear is largely unwarranted. Nearly all cancer-related pain—whether from the disease itself or from surgery and other treatments—can be controlled. Such pain is typically treated with medication taken orally. If you can't take pills or liquids by mouth, other methods can be used to deliver pain medication. Your pain-control plan may utilize many sources of relief.

Pain is complex. You may have a different kind of pain than someone else with exactly the same condition. Why? Pain is always affected by many factors—not just your nerve fibers, but your past experiences with pain and your current physical and emotional state. Do not be surprised if you develop pain from several sources throughout your treatment—from the cancer itself, from mood changes, from treatment, from side effects, and even from some medications.

Cancer-Related Pain

Cancer itself may cause many different degrees of pain depending on the cancer's location. Cancer treatments can cause painful side effects, some of which can be anticipated—for example, pain can be expected at a surgical incision site or in healthy tissues that have been

Learn some relaxing techniques. Let your mind take you out of the treatment room.

Pat, 72
Cancer survivor

damaged by radiation. Other pain may arise unexpectedly. For example, combining radiation with surgery or chemotherapy can cause muscle scarring, which generates a dull ache associated with tensing muscles of the neck or throat.

Whether your pain comes from your cancer or your treatment, it is especially important to not delay pain medication. It should always be taken at the first sign of pain because this maximizes its effectiveness. If possible, it should be taken before the onset of pain. In other words, don't "chase" the pain. Stay ahead of it.

Identifying Pain and Its Severity

The kind of medication used for your pain and how it is administered will depend on what is causing the pain and whether it has more than one cause. It's important that you communicate details of your pain to your physician; doctors and nurses have many tools and techniques for managing your pain, but you need to tell them everything you can. If you think you know what is causing a particular pain, say so. Patients often have good intuition about what is happening in their bodies.

You may also find it helpful to keep a pain diary. Every day, write down everything you can about your pain—even if it is mild or lasts only a short time. Keep track of the following:

- When the pain starts
- Where it is located
- Whether it interferes with movement or function

- Whether it moves around or remains in one place
- What the pain feels like (sharp, dull, throbbing, achy, tingling, burning)
- Whether the pain is constant or whether it comes and goes
- When it is worse—at what times of day and under what conditions (for example, when you are active, when you lie down, after you have eaten, when you press on the affected area)
- Whether you are able to ease it yourself
- The severity of the pain

The severity of your pain is perhaps the most important thing to communicate because it determines which category of medication your doctor will prescribe. To describe your degree of pain, use a scale from 1 to 10, with 1 being mild discomfort to 10 being unbearable pain. If you are having trouble speaking, draw this scale on paper and circle the number between 1 and 10 that applies to your degree of pain.

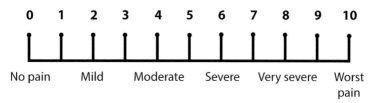

Be sure to keep your medical staff informed about the severity of your pain so they can treat it accordingly. Use this pain scale as a guide to reporting the level of your pain to your health-care team.

Why Pain Can Be Undertreated

An opioid epidemic currently is affecting our country. This has heightened awareness among patients and physicians about the proper use of narcotic pain medication. Many patients have a fear of becoming addicted to narcotics. However, most patients who take medications as directed do not become addicted. Still, many patients are often reluctant to take pain medication for the following reasons.

- Reluctance to report pain, out of concern for sounding like a "complainer"
- Desire for physicians to focus on treating the cancer, not pain
- Fear that pain means the cancer is getting worse
- Fear of addiction or serious side effects

Doctors are learning that there are many ways to relieve pain that may not require narcotics. In addition to using narcotics, most postsurgical pain can be managed with non-narcotic pain medications and ice.

Planning for Pain Control

It is important for you and your physician to develop a plan for pain control before a treatment begins. If you are scheduled for surgery, don't wait to talk to your doctor about pain management until immediately after your operation, when you are groggy. Talk to your doctor ahead of surgery about a plan for pain management.

Your doctor can help you understand what to expect in the way of pain, based on your treatment plan. You, in turn, can give the doctor detailed information about the pain as it occurs. This will determine whether your pain comes from your cancer or from the effects of treatment, and your medications can be managed accordingly.

The constant exchange of information with your doctors is important to your recovery. Patients who are well informed about pain and have good communication with their caregivers report less pain, use less medication, and leave the hospital earlier than those who do not. Reporting any changes in your pain helps your physician adjust medications and dosages as soon as possible.

The following guidelines are important in any pain-control plan, but most apply primarily to postsurgical and treatment-related pain:

- Make sure you and your doctor agree about the importance of managing your pain at every phase of diagnosis and treatment. Ask about your doctor's approach to pain control.
- Describe your worries, concerns, and any pain-control methods that have worked for you in the past.
- Report any pain you experience at any time. Be sure to describe the pain in detail.
- Find out whether your hospital has a specialized pain service that you can call on if your pain is not controlled by routine treatments.
- Begin taking pain medications as soon as pain begins—or sooner, if you know it is likely to occur.
- Ask your doctor about increasing your dose of pain medications before engaging in activities that can worsen pain, such as walking again after surgery.

Medications for Pain

Medications that directly relieve pain are called *analgesics.* There are many kinds of analgesics, and their use is the most common method of controlling nearly all pain. These analgesics are used for pain control:

- Narcotics
- Non-narcotics
- Temporary nerve blocks

Another class of drugs—*antidepressants* and *tran-quilizers*—relieves pain by easing the emotional stresses than can intensify it. These drugs also have a direct analgesic affect.

Narcotics

Narcotics are powerful drugs that work in the brain to block pain throughout the central nervous system. Narcotics such as morphine, codeine, hydrocodone, and hydromorphone are available only by prescription and are used only for severe pain over short periods of time. For patients with severe long-term pain, combinations of therapies are used, sometimes with narcotics or injections for nerve blocks.

Receiving Narcotics while Hospitalized

While you're hospitalized, *patient-controlled analgesia (PCA)* may be used to manage postsurgical pain. This involves having an IV tube attached to a pump that controls the release of narcotic medication. When you have pain, you press a button to release medication through the IV. To prevent an overdose, the pump is regulated to limit the amount of the drug that can be administered over a period of time.

PCA is often used in hospitals because it is easier and more effective than having a nurse give a narcotic by injection. A doctor will determine whether PCA is appropriate based on a patient's general health, his or her ability to follow directions, and the amount of pain that is likely to occur. Fortunately, most operations of the head and neck result in mild to moderate pain that is well controlled without the use of a PCA pump; postsurgical pain often does not require narcotic use.

Narcotics can be given in pill form or as a liquid, either orally or through a nasal or stomach tube. They can also be delivered with a patch applied to the skin, by injection, or through an IV tube or an *epidural*—a small tube placed in the spine. A skin patch is especially good for providing a constant dose of medication—especially a low dose over a longer period of time. The patch is an alternative for people who have trouble swallowing pills or liquids.

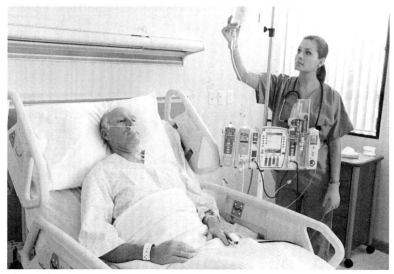

Patient-controlled analgesia (PCA) is delivered through an IV. To receive more pain medication, a patient presses a button. The machine is set so it cannot deliver too much medication. *Photo courtesy and copyright Becton, Dickinson, and Company.*

Narcotic Side Effects

Narcotics nearly always produce drowsiness or sedation, which can actually be beneficial because they can help you get the rest you need. Other possible side effects are constipation, itching, bladder irregularity, vivid dreams, and nausea. Most people get used to the nausea, but if it is severe, other medications can bring the nausea under control.

Non-Narcotics

Several common nonprescription medications are used to treat surgical and cancer-related pain. These include acetaminophen (such as *Tylenol*), aspirin, and ibuprofen (such as *Advil* and *Motrin*). Acetaminophen relieves pain and fever but does not reduce inflammation. Aspirin and ibuprofen, which belong to a category of medications called *nonsteroidal anti-inflammatory drugs (NSAIDs),* relieve pain, fever, and inflammation.

Cox II inhibitors is a category of anti-inflammatory drugs. *Celebrex* is an example. These drugs have all the same effects as other non-narcotic pain medications, but they tend to generate less stomach upset and may temporarily decrease the ability of the blood to form clots, prolonging bleeding from injuries.

All of these non-narcotics control pain at its source,whereas the narcotics control pain through the central nervous system. Non-narcotics are the first line of medication pain control and often are all that is required. They can be used over long periods of time because they do not cause dependency.

Non-Narcotic Side Effects

Aspirin and NSAIDs can inflame the stomach lining and can also reduce the blood's clotting ability, which may result in prolonged bleeding from injuries. Also, individuals preparing for surgery may not want to take these medications because they thin the blood and promote bleeding. Talk to your doctor well in advance of your surgery if you are taking these drugs to determine if stopping these medications is appropriate before your surgery.

Nerve Blocks

When severe pain is highly localized—for example, at a surgical incision—it can sometimes be controlled by temporarily blocking the nerves at the site. This is done by injecting a local anesthetic such as *Xylocaine* or *bupivacaine*. There are no significant side effects to this method, and it can reduce the need for narcotics in the short term.

Permanent nerve blocks can also be used for more chronic, or long-term, localized pain. In this case—if a pain specialist determines the procedure is appropriate— the nerve in question is injected with a local anesthetic. If that relieves the pain, the nerve can then be injected with a substance that will destroy it. This leaves the affected area numb, and it usually significantly diminishes or eliminates the pain. However, this procedure is invasive, and it carries a risk of unexpected outcomes, including no pain relief at all or even increased pain.

Tranquilizers and Antidepressants

If anxiety or depression contributes to your pain, you doctor may recommend adding a tranquilizer or an antidepressant to your medication regimen. The calming effects of these drugs not only can help reduce pain but also can help you sleep and function better.

Antidepressants prescribed today include such drugs as *Prozac, Celexa,* or *Lexapro*; they are also effective for chronic pain. Side effects of all antidepressants may include temporary sedation and drowsiness.

Patients who have been taking antidepressants for some time will want to have their physicians guide them in gradually tapering off the antidepressants, rather than stopping abruptly. The tapering helps avoid a sudden return of depression symptoms.

An older class of antidepressants called *tricyclics* are especially beneficial for patients suffering chronic pain. They are used both alone and in combination with other medications.

Other Pain-Control Methods

Surgical and cancer-related pain can be often be relieved by methods that do not involve medications. When pain is severe, these methods are often used along with medications, sometimes reinforcing their beneficial effects. When pain is mild or moderate, these other methods can sometimes be used instead of any medication at all.

TENS Unit

A *transcutaneous electrical nerve-stimulation unit (TENS)* treats pain without medication. The TENS unit is a small electrical box, about the size of a deck of cards, that can be attached to a belt; electrodes connected to the box are applied to the area where you experience pain. The device works by sending low-level electrical currents across the skin and blocking pain signals from reaching the brain. This method has very few side effects except for minor skin irritation. The only drawback is that it can lose effectiveness as your nerves adapt to it.

Physical Therapy

When muscles are damaged or weakened by surgery and other therapies, physical therapy can often do wonders to reduce pain and restore strength and flexibility. If your doctor orders physical therapy, you will also be given a series of stretching and strengthening exercises to do daily, either on your own or with a physical therapist's help. You might also be instructed to apply cold packs (usually for swelling) or heat packs, either moist or dry. You will be warned against using heat on areas where you have numbness. Why? Because if you don't feel sensation in the area, the danger of burns is always high, especially if you use a microwave oven to warm your heat packs.

9

Coping Emotionally

A diagnosis of cancer can unleash strong emotions. Most cancer patients are flooded with emotions—fear, anger, anxiety, and sadness. These emotions are not signs of weakness. They are normal reactions. These feelings are often so overwhelming that denial—a refusal to accept or deal with the new reality—may initially keep them at bay until the mind can gradually adjust to the news.

A diagnosis of cancer can turn a person's life upside down. However, if your emotions do not gradually ease up—and especially if they get worse—they can interfere with concentration, sleep, appetite, and your ability to follow a treatment plan. This can interfere with your body's ability to heal and your mind's ability to grasp the information you will need to make important decisions.

Stress and Depression

Negative emotions can impede treatment in other ways, too. Prolonged psychological stress appears to undermine the immune system. It has long been known that painful, life-changing events such as divorce, the loss of a job, or a death in the family can increase a person's risk of illness. Research studies have shown that chronic stress can impair the ability of cells to repair themselves, a condition that could influence the development and progress of cancer. Other studies indicate that excessive amounts of stress-related hormones might weaken the immune system; high stress levels also create a posttraumatic stress situation that can cause long-term changes to the emotional centers of the brain, especially during radiation therapy.

One out of three individuals becomes depressed while undergoing cancer treatment, especially if they receive radiation therapy to the head or neck. Studies suggest that use of an antidepressant prior to starting such treatment may prevent depression and improve quality of life. Ask your doctor if you might benefit from an antidepressant. These drugs are not addictive, and you and your doctor may choose to discontinue them later on.

Coping Strategies

A cancer diagnosis, like any sudden, frightening event, can make you feel as if you have lost all control over your life. That is why it is important to identify areas in which you still can make decisions and exert your influence.

There are many steps you can take to ease the shock of your diagnosis and cope with the emotional turmoil it will create for a while. For example, minimizing other stresses in your life will free your energies for the important challenges ahead of you. It will improve your ability to understand your illness, make informed choices about your treatment, and find new ways to care for your health and well-being. Following are some ways of coping with stress.

Positive "Self-Talk"

Because many cancers of the mouth and throat result from the use of tobacco, mostly smoking, many individuals feel guilty for having cancer. They believe they caused the cancer. They blame and berate themselves. Even though a cancer may have resulted from a lifestyle habit, now is a time to be loving and gentle with yourself.

If you find yourself dealing with self-blame, remind yourself that you may have used tobacco for a variety of reasons, none of which included the intention to get cancer. Remind yourself that addictions are powerful forces, and the strongest of people find them difficult to break.

An individual who has a cancer that is associated with HPV also may have a range of emotions and concerns about their partner. The individual may worry that their partner will "catch" the cancer. This is not the case. The virus that caused the cancer is virtually always gone by the time the individual develops the cancer. These infections usually have occurred many years, even decades, prior to the actual cancer being detected.

Taking Care of Yourself Emotionally

Just knowing where your emotional "hot spots" are can help you cope. Do you find yourself always trying to please others rather than doing what is right for you? For example, do you find it hard to say no when you're asked to help others? Do you readily take on new assignments in your work? Do you belong to clubs or organizations that hold frequent meetings and keep you out at night? Do your extracurricular activities drain you or give you energy?

It is important to examine such questions early in your treatment. You must put your emotional and physical health first—before your job, your community commitments, and even family responsibilities. Of course, you won't want to give up family responsibilities or your contacts with friends, but you can let *them* help *you* with things you have previously taken on. You probably won't give up your job, either, but perhaps you can delegate tasks, take advantage of any vacation time or sick time, and find other ways to lighten your workload.

After diagnosis of cancer of the voice box, I thought treatment had to begin immediately. My doctor reassured me that my cancer did not spread that fast and that waiting two to three weeks was okay.

Ron, 64
Cancer survivor

None of this is selfish. Eliminating whatever exhausting or stressful activities you can is simply necessary. In general, you should avoid tasks, people, and situations that tax your patience and energy. Seek out those that inspire you, give you strength, and make you feel good about yourself.

Reaching Out to Others

The broader your social network, the more people you will be able to draw on for strength and support. Affectionate bonds bring comfort, and they make a person feel worthwhile. Be prepared for some people to feel awkward, though. Many will not know how to talk with you about your illness, or whether they should even try. Their own fears, whether of losing you, upsetting you, or facing their own mortality, might intrude on their best intentions.

You, too, may have avoided any discussion of the topics that are now interrupting your life—topics such as illness, pain, loss, or death. So think about your relationships, and ask yourself who is most likely to help you and welcome your efforts to open up. Who is the best listener? Who knows the territory you are entering, having already been through a major illness? Whom do you trust the most? Who would help you with your daily activities, either at work or at home? Your family, friends, and coworkers will probably feel relieved and encouraged if you can tell them what you need from them.

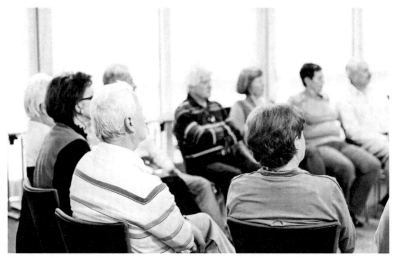

Support groups offer a safe place to express emotions with others who are experiencing similar issues. You can share as much or as little as you wish; these groups can be very comforting.

Nutrition, Sleep, and Exercise

Good nutrition promotes the body's ability to heal. Plenty of rest eases tension, helps a person cope with emotionally difficult situations, and also gives the body an opportunity to repair itself. Moderate, regular exercise—within the bounds of your condition—stimulates the cardiovascular system and tones muscles. It also reduces the amount of stress hormones in your body and releases other hormones, called *endorphins,* that promote a sense of well-being. Exercising outdoors in good weather and pleasant surroundings further enhances mood.

Meditation and Relaxation

Any exercise or routine that calms the mind and creates a contemplative, relaxed mood is beneficial in emotionally difficult times. Deep relaxation techniques are valuable, too, especially those that focus the mind on positive thoughts or on the gradual easing of tight muscles and emotional tension. For example, mindfulness and meditation soothe the mind and often generate images of healing and hope. Deep, slow abdominal breathing, practiced several times a day, can sensitize you to parts of the body in which stress accumulates and can gradually help you relax them, promoting a feeling of peace.

There are a great many ways to relax your mind and body. Listening to music might do it for some; painting or meditative dance might do it for others. Finding a method that works for you, one that you can sustain throughout your treatment, is one of the best things you can do for yourself.

Massages, Embraces, Pets

Any gentle contact with another warm body can work wonders in reducing distress and anxiety. A hug from a friend can ease loneliness or fears of burdening others. A shoulder rub from a mate both relieves tense muscles and communicates love. A full-body massage in a spa or health club deeply relaxes the body and promotes a sense of serenity. Studies even show that having a pet, especially one that responds to caresses with affection, offers similar benefits. If you have never been a very physically expressive person, now may be the time to experience the delights of becoming one.

Getting Professional Help

What if you can't control your fearful emotions and anxieties on your own? What if your fears, depression, or anger are taking a toll on you? There is value in some of these uncomfortable emotions. Every form of distress that follows a cancer diagnosis may serve a purpose. For example, denial can give you some time to adjust to the idea of having cancer. Anger, especially when it is directed at the cancer, can pump you up with energy and determination. Sadness can provide release, lessening tensions. Even self-blame, in moderation, can give you an

My surgeon encouraged me to get a second opinion because I was confused and angry about having cancer. I liked my doctor and had confidence in him, but it was reassuring to hear someone else tell me the same things my first doctor told me.

Seth, 42
Cancer patient

opportunity to assess your life honestly and allow you to forgive your all-too-human errors.

But these same emotions can become prolonged and have a destructive effect on you. Denial can keep you from learning what you need to know about your cancer and its treatment. You may turn anger toward your caregivers or even your family. Sadness can deepen into clinical depression. Self-blame can even convince you that you deserve to have cancer.

It is important that you talk with your doctor if your emotions feel out of control. Any number of things can dangerously prolong the emotional difficulties caused by your diagnosis. The following are just a few situations that could call for therapy:

- You have recently suffered a serious loss, moved away from your community, or faced family or financial problems.

- You feel guilty about your cancer, either because you fear you will burden your loved ones or because you feel you caused your illness by smoking, excessive alcohol use, overworking, or other lifestyle choices.

- You encounter blaming or judgmental attitudes in others.

- You have a history of depression, poor self-esteem, or a tendency to avoid problems rather than facing them.

- It is your habit to "go it alone," keeping your feelings and needs bottled up when you really would feel better finding ways to express them.

Do not worry about being perceived as a complainer when you seek help for your emotional state. It is important to open up, even if you are not used to doing so, even if you have always managed your life without much help from others. If your doctor doesn't ask you the kinds of questions that will help you talk about your anxieties, you should raise them yourself or ask for a referral to a mental health professional. This is especially important if you experience any of the following:

- Anxiety attacks
- Inability to sleep, eat, or concentrate
- Persistent feelings of worthlessness
- Preoccupation with death or suicide
- Significant weight gain or weight loss
- Loss of interest in your usual activities
- Loss of interest in sex

Sometimes these are signs of a serious psychological disturbance or an undiagnosed medical condition. Sometimes they are side effects of medications. Your doctor needs to determine the underlying cause and then help you decide whether to seek professional counseling or a psychiatric evaluation. You might choose individual psychotherapy, group therapy, a support group, or family therapy. Any of these, together or in combination, can help you improve your quality of life and your ability to cope.

Seeking therapy is not a sign of weakness, nor is a stiff upper lip always a sign of strength. When you suppress your emotions, you intensify the stress your body must absorb. When you express your feelings constructively—rather than by lashing out against yourself or others—you minimize your stress. If your relationships with others already are conflicted, so that free and honest emotional expression is hampered, therapy can often help open the channels of communication. It can also teach you how to assert yourself, look after your own interests, and participate fully in every decision you face, from treatment options to ways of handling your personal and financial affairs. Remember: part of being independent is knowing when to ask for help.

Regaining Control

The sooner you gain sufficient emotional perspective to begin learning about your illness and treatment options, the sooner you will experience the power that information and action can bring about. The more you know, the more actively you can participate in decisions affecting your treatment. Talk with your doctors. Read everything you can find about your cancer. Ask questions. Learn from other patients and survivors. As you come to understand the kind of cancer you have and your treatment options at every step, your feelings of helplessness will diminish.

10

CLINICAL TRIALS

Cancer patients often turn to experimental therapies when standard treatments have not managed to shrink or eliminate their cancers. Essentially, all drugs introduced in the United States over the past fifty years were experimental at one time.

By joining research studies that test new treatments, many patients turn discouragement into new hope. These studies, called *clinical trials,* are launched only after the new treatments have already been tested extensively in laboratories. If testing indicates that the experimental therapies appear to be at least as good as standard therapies, with the potential to be even better, the treatment is made available to patients. Such trials give patients access to the most recent and promising advances. The treatments may include new drugs, radiation techniques, surgical approaches, and combinations and sequences of treatment, including gene therapy.

However, when experimental therapies are used in cases that have previously failed to improve with standard treatment, they seldom result in a cure. Nevertheless, these experimental therapies at times can result in life extension of a year or more and may also bring improvement in symptoms.

Still, sometimes a patient may be cured with experimental therapy, so hope is not irrational. Other times, the clinical trials have positive results, but the benefits are more modest. Symptoms may be eased or the tumor may shrink or even disappear temporarily.

How Do Clinical Trials Work?

Clinical trials take place in a variety of settings. *Investigator-initiated trials* are usually conducted at universities to test therapies originated by a single researcher or team. The trials are usually small and each represents a one-of-a-kind opportunity for patients to obtain a treatment not available through any other studies. In this type of trial, participants are generally from the area where the trial is being conducted.

Cooperative group trials are supervised by a single organization but are run at numerous cancer centers, clinics, hospitals, and even doctors' offices. Several organizations have been formed just to oversee trials of this kind. Large cooperative groups such as NRG Oncology and Cancer Research Network and other organizations exist only to test new therapies or combinations of therapies in multicenter settings and to disseminate information about their study results. They are usually funded through the National Cancer Institutes (NCI) to compare standard and experimental treatments for common cancers. Cooperative group trials are also used to test therapies for very rare cancers. Because these trials are run at many different locations, they are able to find and treat enough test subjects to obtain reliable results.

Finally, pharmaceutical companies also sponsor clinical trials of new cancer drugs in order to satisfy Food and Drug Administration (FDA) requirements for extensive testing before the new drugs can be marketed. These industry-based trials are held at community cancer centers, hospitals, universities, and doctors' offices. The trials are overseen by the drug companies but the actual testing is performed by individual physicians. For example, a patient who has given his or her consent may

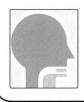

It made me feel good to participate in a clinical trial, knowing that I might be helping someone else with cancer.

Sarah, 33
Cancer patient

receive an injection of a known drug in a novel manner: the injection will be given by the patient's own physician at a hospital; results will be forwarded to the sponsoring drug company for analysis.

Monitoring

Regardless of where clinical trials are held, patients' interests and the need for reliable outcomes must always outweigh other priorities. Researchers sometimes stand to profit from their discoveries, either financially or professionally, and institutions likewise can have a stake in a successful trial. Thus, careful oversight is required at every step of a trial to ensure that these motives remain secondary.

The first step in a clinical trial, once laboratory testing has shown promise for a new drug or therapy, is for participating researchers and doctors to write a *protocol,* or treatment plan. This spells out exactly what therapy is going to be tested, how and in what dosages it will be delivered and monitored, how many patients will participate, how long the study will take, where it will be conducted, and which controls and safeguards will be used.

Controls are especially important. The controls are techniques for ensuring that test results are accurate—that the outcomes of clinical trials are truly the result of the therapy being tested and not some other factor, such as smoking or alcohol intake, exercise, or overall health.

Once a protocol has been drafted, it must be submitted to an *institutional review board (IRB)* for approval before the clinical trial can proceed. IRB members are usually representatives of the general public (such as clergy, teachers, lawyers, and others interested in committing large amounts of time to reviewing protocols), as well as doctors and researchers who have no personal or professional stake in the trial.

The IRB monitors the clinical trial from beginning to end to make sure that it follows strict ethical standards. These standards are outlined in part by the federal government and the international community. In turn, the FDA and the Office of Protection from Research Risks (OPRR) periodically review the conduct of the IRB. These measures ensure the quality of the testing, the welfare of participating patients, and the priorities of the researchers and doctors.

The IRB will also review the *informed consent,* a document that must be signed by every patient who takes part in the trial. It explains the nature of the study and any expected side effects, risks, health benefits, payments, or costs that might be involved. Usually the cost of the drug is covered by insurance or by the trial sponsor, but routine laboratory analysis and radiographs may not be covered.

Phases of Clinical Trials

Clinical trials typically take place in four phases. The purpose of a Phase I trial is to determine the safest dose or delivery method for a treatment and to pay close attention to any side effects it produces. Most people who enroll in a Phase I trial have either not responded to standard treatments or are unlikely to benefit from them.

A Phase II trial, conducted after the best dosage or treatment method has been determined, tests whether the new therapy is effective in decreasing the size of a cancer. Researchers hope to see 20 to 30 percent of participants responding favorably with tumor shrinkage or disappearance.

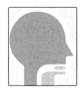

We were all a little nervous when dad's doctors wanted him to participate in a clinical trial. We did not want our dad on some experimental drug. It was reassuring to know what kinds of research and studies had already been done to get to this stage.

Sally, 32
Daughter of cancer patient

After a treatment has proven effective in an acceptable percentage of cases with acceptable side effects, it proceeds to a Phase III trial, where it is compared with standard treatments. Reliable results in Phase III require many more participants than other phases. In general, Phase III trials consist of one group to which standard therapies are given and one to which the experimental therapies are given.

To make sure the two groups can be compared equally, participants must meet detailed eligibility requirements. Some trials enroll only previously untreated patients, whereas others require patients for whom radiation and surgery have already failed. The groups are then matched for age, sex, general health status, tobacco and alcohol use, and other factors deemed important to ensuring comparable groups for study. After patients have been selected for the trial, they are randomly assigned to either the standard or the experimental group. Typically, half the patients in a randomized trial will not receive an experimental drug.

Usually, the FDA approves a drug or treatment if the first three phases of clinical testing produce favorable results. However, continued testing and monitoring are required even after the therapy is in widespread use. This later testing constitutes a Phase IV trial, and it documents the new therapy's efficacy and safety in even larger groups of patients. This trial shows how the new therapy works in the real world with many patients that might not have been eligible for the initial trials due to health issues or age. This final phase is needed because it's possible that misleading results can arise even from large Phase III trials, and rechecking the data is a further safeguard.

Not every clinical trial will require all four phases of testing. Sometimes, a trial ends early when a treatment results in clearly superior standard treatments. In contrast, the trial may not proceed if the treatment results are inferior or the treatment produces unacceptable side effects.

Taking Part in a Clinical Trial

If you think you might be eligible for a clinical trial, your doctor can help you identify one that is appropriate for you. He or she will review with you every detail of the trial's protocol and will then ask you to sign an informed consent; this document confirms your awareness of risks, benefits, procedures, and possible costs or payments to you. Before you enroll or sign the consent form, ask your doctor the following questions:

- Am I eligible for the trial? What are the criteria for joining?
- How does the new therapy being tested in the trial differ from the treatments I have already received?
- How might the new therapy improve on the standard therapies?
- What risks might arise if I participate? What benefits?
- How long will the treatment take? Will I have to be away from home?
- Will my insurance cover the full cost of tests and procedures in the trial?

After you join a trial, your participation is voluntary at each phase. You may withdraw at any time before, during, or after receiving the experimental treatment.

Whether you complete the trial or not, you will receive medical care for any problems that may result from your participation. However, you may be responsible for the costs of such treatment.

Advantages of Clinical Trials

- You receive therapy that has been tested in laboratories and appears to be at least as good as standard therapies.
- You are among the first to receive the new therapy.
- The new therapy may succeed where standard treatments have not.
- Your responses to the new treatment will be monitored closely by doctors who specialize in cancer therapy.
- Your participation may help in the development of cancer therapies that will benefit others in the future.

Disadvantages of Clinical Trials

- The new therapy may not prove more effective than standard treatments; it could even be less effective.
- You could experience unexpected, or unexpectedly severe, side effects.
- You may be responsible for costs not covered by your insurance.
- You may need to travel a significant distance to participate if the new treatment is not being tested at a location near you.

In Summary

Patients are often willing to participate in clinical trials in the hope that the experimental therapies might help both themselves and others in the future. This is how progress is made in cancer treatment.

To find a clinical trial, visit the U.S. National Library of Medicine website at www.clinicaltrials.gov. This site provides a database of privately and publically funded clinical trials being conducted around the world.

PART III

AFTER TREATMENT

Clear and Cool
December 2

Walking in darkness,
beneath a billion indifferent stars
at quarter to six in the morning,
the moon already down
and gone, but keeping a pale lamp burning
at the edge of the west,
my shoes too loud in the gravel
that, faintly lit, looks to be little more
than a contrail of vapor,
so thin, so insubstantial it could,
on a whim, let me drop through it
and out of the day.
But I have taught myself
to place one foot ahead of the other
in noisy confidence
as if each morning might be trusted,
as if the sounds I make might buoy me up.

—*Ted Kooser*
Poet Laureate
of the United States
(2004–2005)

11

FOLLOW-UP CARE

Once your cancer treatments have ended, follow-up care is important. Depending on your type of cancer and treatment, your doctor will likely want to follow up with you on a regular basis for several years.

Doctor Visits

For the first one or two years after your treatment has ended, you will need to see your doctor every two to three months, to make sure you have no signs of a new or recurring cancer. By five years, if you have remained cancer-free, you will need a follow-up visit only once or twice a year.

If your cancer is still present, follow-up will likely take place every four to eight weeks. In this case, the major purpose is to assess pain control, help with nutrition, provide emotional support, and keep the communication channels open.

Above all, be sure to keep your scheduled follow-up appointments. Follow-up visits serve three vital purposes:

- *Early detection.* This is most important of all, since new or recurring cancers and precancerous conditions can be treated most successfully if they are caught right away.

- *Relief.* In most cases, there is no new or recurring cancer, and this good news can be a boost to the spirits.
- *Communication.* These visits are opportunities to talk with your doctor about your emotional and physical well-being, your progress with rehabilitation, and any questions you've had on your mind.

One question you might want to raise in your follow-up visits is whether your doctor can suggest ways to alleviate any remaining side effects of your treatment. New therapies are always being developed. For side effects that can't be cured—including some forms of disfigurement and the need for artificial speech—you might find it helpful to talk with other patients, individually or in a support group. Or you might ask your doctor to recommend a counselor.

Don't Wait to See Your Doctor

Remember, any time you have a problem or a troubling symptom, you should see your doctor immediately. Don't wait until your next scheduled appointment. Some patients find this hard to do; many patients feel great anxiety before a follow-up visit, worrying about the possibility of facing either a new cancer or the spread of any cancer that has remained in the body.

It is true that someone who has already had cancer is at higher risk than someone who has not. Still, your risk of developing a new, primary cancer is about 2 to 4 percent per year, so it remains relatively unlikely that this particular fear will become reality. It is difficult to predict a rate of cancer recurrence, since it depends on the original stage and location of a cancer.

It is equally important to detect precancerous conditions so that they can be prevented from becoming cancers. Such conditions can include mouth lesions, or sore spots, called *leukoplakia* (white patches) and *erythropla-*

What is important to me is to maintain an active social life. Being able to attend church, school functions, go out to eat in nice restaurants, and to be able to go fishing.

V.L., 74
Mouth cancer survivor

sia (red patches). Lesions can be removed in a variety of ways and the cells examined for abnormalities. Treatment depends on the results of cell analysis. For example, if *dysplastic cells* are found (that is, cells that show abnormal growth but are not yet cancerous), treatment usually requires removal with a laser, excision, or the topical application of a chemotherapy medication.

If cell analysis shows an increase in *keratin* (the kind of horny tissue found in hair and nails), this, too, is a danger sign, though a mild one, which becomes cancerous less than 5 percent of the time. Depending on the location of the cells, this condition usually requires patients to quit smoking, to have dentures refitted, or to remove other irritants.

You should know which symptoms to look out for in particular. A red patch is more likely to turn cancerous than a white one. A lump of tissue is much more worrisome than a soft, flat area. But any abnormal growth in the mouth or neck should be checked immediately—especially any lump in the neck that develops along with a sore in the mouth. Surprisingly, cancer in its early stages usually does not cause pain. Therefore small, painful mouth ulcers, like canker sores, are seldom malignant.

Giving Up Tobacco

Every cancer survivor worries that their disease will come back—but much can be done to minimize that worry. In the case of mouth and throat cancer, especially, there is an obvious and effective means of prevention: quit smoking. In fact, quit using tobacco in any form.

Perhaps you have stopped using tobacco. Your doctors will have urged you to do so even before starting your treatment, to reduce both a chance of cancer recurrence or the development of a new cancer.

However, giving up tobacco is no simple matter. Nicotine is very addictive. When you smoke, nicotine is sent to your brain. A chemical called *dopamine* is released, making you feel good. Then, when your dopamine levels drop, it makes you want to smoke again.

Add to that the fact that you might have started smoking decades ago. By now, you have a whole set of deep-seated habits to break—smoking to calm your nerves, smoking to relieve boredom, smoking just for the pleasure of it. Perhaps your friends or spouse smoke, too, so you encounter tobacco and smoke nearly everywhere you go. Perhaps you fear that if you quit you will gain a lot of weight—though, for most cancer patients, weight gain should be a goal, not a thing to avoid. Ask yourself which of these obstacles lie in your way when you think about quitting tobacco. Then develop a strategy to minimize or overcome them.

Review Risks

You already know the risks of tobacco use: heart attack, stroke, cancer, emphysema, other respiratory illnesses, and the hazards of secondary smoke for your loved ones. You have already suffered one of the most serious consequences of smoking, and there is no stronger motivation than the desire not to face that consequence again. No matter how serious or long-standing your addiction, take the matter of quitting one day—or even one hour—at a time. This way, your motivation will stay strong, and your motivation is the most important factor in quitting.

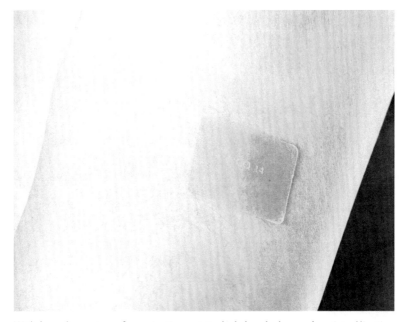

Withdrawal symptoms from nicotine may include headaches and anxiety. Nicotine patches, worn on the upper arm, reduce cravings for cigarettes.

Plan for Smoking Cessation

Start by giving up tobacco for just twenty-four hours. This short time is a long step toward beating your addiction. If you can quit for just one day, you'll be able to quit for just one more day—and keep on doing that, one day at a time.

In the meantime, look for ways to make the challenge easier. Avoid as many "triggers" for smoking as you can— perhaps long telephone conversations, lingering over a cup of coffee, feeling stressed. If you can't avoid anxiety, try deep breathing or meditation instead of smoking. Find a partner—someone else who is quitting, with whom you can share support. Some cancer centers have smoking support groups, much like Alcoholics Anonymous, and these use both the buddy system and any necessary medical means. Above all, ask your doctor for help. He or she can prescribe medications and can help you locate support groups and other resources.

Anti-Smoking Medications

Anti-smoking medications are available. Perhaps you've heard of the "nicotine patch," a widely advertised and successful means of helping people quit smoking. The patch uses nicotine to fight the nicotine addiction. The patch is worn against the skin to deliver nicotine in continuous but steadily decreasing doses over time. This allows smokers to wean themselves gradually from their need for nicotine.

Nicotine gum and spray are also used for this purpose. They give a quick burst of nicotine when the urge becomes strong. The gum and patch can be obtained over the counter. The nasal and aerosol nicotine sprays require a prescription from your doctor. Sometimes patients use the patch in combination with the gum or spray, but this should be done with a doctor's supervision. Depending on how much you smoke, the cost of these useful nicotine delivery systems could be less than the cost of tobacco. In any case, over time, this approach will be far less expensive than continued tobacco use.

Some people give up tobacco with the help of a drug called *Zyban,* with the active component bupropion. Most patients start by taking the drug once a day for three days, then increase the dose to twice a day. They pick a quit date ten to fourteen days from the first dose. During the period before the quit date, tobacco is likely to stop tasting good, and desire for it will diminish. Sometimes, Zyban also reduces addiction symptoms. You may need to stay on this medicine for three months or more in order to stay off tobacco for good.

Another prescription drug, *Chantix,* may also help you quit smoking. This drug blocks the effects of nicotine on your brain so that you don't feel the same urge to smoke. Talk to your physician about whether one of these drugs might be helpful.

Giving Up Alcohol

Limiting alcohol intake may also reduce the risk of cancer. Although there is clearly a cancer risk from any tobacco use, there is less evidence of any risk from moderate alcohol use—no more than two drinks a day. Heavy alcohol use is another matter. If you routinely consume more than five drinks per day, you should simply quit drinking. Any alcohol use in combination with tobacco is especially harmful. The combination increases the risk for cancer by forty times in heavy drinkers and smokers.

As with tobacco, the first step is a desire to quit. If you believe you need help quitting, you might wish to consider a support group such as Alcoholics Anonymous; it has helped millions accomplish this challenge. Research shows that it is difficult to recover from alcoholism by yourself. Support groups can offer education and support for giving up alcohol.

A note about surgery and drinking. If you are about to undergo surgery and decide to quit drinking all at once, make sure your doctors are aware of your usual alcohol intake because withdrawal from alcohol can produce *delirium tremens,* or *DTs.* This is a short-term condition, but it can be fatal if it is not treated with drugs that ease the withdrawal symptoms.

Even if you don't have a drinking problem, it is always a good idea to limit your alcohol intake after cancer treatment. One or two drinks a day is probably all right, unless your doctor recommends you not drink. If you are an alcoholic, or have poor nutrition or mouth sores, your doctor will probably recommend that you not use any alcohol at all.

Good Nutrition

From the very beginning of their illnesses, many people with mouth or throat cancer find it difficult to eat or swallow because of painful tumors. In addition, the cancer increases the metabolic demands on the body, meaning that more nutrition is needed to fight the disease. Patients often lose weight and muscle mass even before treatment begins. After treatment is under way, side effects can make the problem worse.

Your doctors want to work with you to maintain your weight. After your treatment has ended, you will need to learn how to manage your diet and keep your weight up on your own. Your continued healing and good health depend on this. But if various cancer treatments have left you with little ability to taste food, or eating is difficult, the formerly simple act of eating can seem an insurmountable challenge. Fortunately, there are ways to address these difficulties. In most cases, your doctor will be able to pinpoint your problem and recommend techniques that can help you eat.

Nutritional Assessment

You might need to have your nutritional plan evaluated. Naturally, the first indicator is your weight. If it is 10 percent or more below your normal weight, there is cause for concern. Blood tests, too, can indicate the quality of your nutrition, by measuring levels of albumen and other proteins. And urine can be tested for nitrogen levels. Nitrogen is produced by the breakdown of protein, and in malnourished patients the protein stored in muscles will break down to meet the body's metabolic demands. This is called a "negative nitrogen balance" and is detrimental to healing. It deprives the muscles of needed fuel and can lead to a loss of muscle mass.

After your nutrition plan has been evaluated, you may need to meet with a nutritionist to work out a plan for maintaining a healthy diet. This person will help you determine your caloric and protein needs and some methods for meeting them. Each day, you will need to weigh yourself, record your weight, and keep track of what you are eating and how much. You might need to take high-calorie, high-protein nutritional supplements, at least for a while. You might also need to eat smaller meals more frequently in order to take in enough nutrients without taxing your ability to eat too much food at once.

Cancer Survivorship Programs

As more people are surviving cancer, survivorship programs are being developed to help them move from cancer patient to cancer survivor. These programs help individuals cope with the physical, psychological, emotional, social, and even spiritual issues that often surface even after successful therapy.

Cancer survivorship programs reflect the fact that a growing number of Americans are disease-free after treatment. National Cancer Institute (NCI) statistics tell us that more than 15.5 million Americans are living with a history of cancer. Other NCI estimates project the number of people surviving beyond their diagnosis will reach 19 million by 2024.

Survivorship programs that support the well-being and unique needs of patients are important additions to the care of head and neck patients.

Challenges after Treatment

Even cancer patients with promising prognoses may have a need for treatment of future medical, psychological, and other issues. For example, cancer or its therapy may cause progressive damage to the swallowing mechanism or to other organs; or, a cancer might recur years later.

The physical after-effects, however, aren't the only concern. More than half of individuals undergoing cancer treatment become depressed at some point during their lives. They also often experience fear that a cancer will return despite intensive treatment. Even reaching a milestone in recovery can trigger doubts and skepticism about the ability to stay healthy. Any physical change or symptom, for example, may raise fears that the cancer is back.

Further, survivors may experience grief over the perceived loss of their health, physical independence, self-esteem, and other aspects of their life. They also may need help in adjusting to possible changes in their relationships with family members, friends, and even coworkers. Since cancer can be an isolating experience, patients often need help in approaching others who avoid them or don't want to talk about their disease. And while they may face guilt over surviving the cancer, they also may experience a renewed sense of spirituality or religious conviction.

Support after Treatment

After cancer treatment, cancer survivorship programs help patients overcome psychological or physical issues by providing expertise, education, and other resources. A team of medical professionals and survivorship specialists help individuals identify their specific challenges and then address them with the necessary tools. That includes therapy for emotional concerns, support groups, classes, family member counseling, and access to community services and professionals.

Even though a survivorship treatment plan is unique to an individual, it will likely include the following:

Regular physical examinations. Patients not only learn to manage possible long-term effects of their disease, but also focus on normal health maintenance in supporting their results. As part of reviewing a patient's overall health, the medical team emphasizes monitoring and screening for both new and recurring cancers.

Management of treatment-related side effects. Even with successful therapy, cancer survivors can experience numbness in the hands and feet along with other

I really did not want to go back for my follow-up care. I was scared that they might find that the cancer was back. My wife would make me go, and I am glad she did. I am still doing well and each visit gives me more confidence.

Dennis, 57
Tongue cancer patient

residual effects that may influence their daily activities. A survivorship program gives patients tools for addressing those and other health problems. Since cancer can also affect preexisting and chronic conditions, working with specialists after treatment can be an important step in addressing any remaining health challenges related to those problems.

Lifestyle coaching. Cancer survivorship programs emphasize changes that boost a person's overall well-being while reducing future cancer risks. By focusing on proper nutrition, exercise, and lifestyle choices, patients gain new tools for maximizing their health as well as continuing their success with treatment. Exercise physiologists and nutritionists are often helpful.

Referrals. Although a patient's primary physicians are still central to care, survivorship programs also offer expert opinions and links to medical specialists with experience working specifically with similar patients in recovery. They can help with fertility, sexual health, and issues related to cancer or treatment. Survivorship programs also can be helpful sources for employment, insurance, and other financial information.

For more information, you may wish to contact The National Coalition for Cancer Survivorship, at their website at www.canceradvocacy.org. By providing a continuum of care, a multidisciplinary team can help patients improve quality of life beyond their cancer treatment.

Lifelong Learning

This chapter offers only some of the information that can help you maintain a good quality of life after your treatment has ended. You can take it from here. Keep exploring and keep learning. Use resources available in your community and in the cancer community at large. Explore the Internet. Rely only on material that is well documented. If you don't have a computer, check your local library, which is likely to have computers linked to the Internet and people who can show you how to get online and search for relevant websites. Stay in touch with your doctor, and don't stop asking questions until you get the resources you feel you need.

The Vernal Equinox
March 20th

How important it must be
to someone
that I am alive, and walking,
and that I have written
these poems.
This morning the sun stood
right at the end of the road
and waited for me.

—*Ted Kooser*
Poet Laureate
of the United States
(2004–2005)

Appendix

Surgeries for Mouth and Throat Cancers

The operations described in the following pages are the most common ones performed for mouth and throat cancers. Higher-stage cancers often require combinations of these operations. Reconstruction operations appear at the end of this appendix.

Tongue and Floor of the Mouth

Surgery: Excision of small premalignant or malignant lesion of the tongue or floor of mouth (early stage, T1 or T2)

Description: The cancerous or precancerous tissue is removed with a margin of normal tissue. Procedure is performed through the mouth, with either local or general anesthesia, usually on an outpatient basis or with an overnight hospital stay.

Reconstruction: Wound is closed with sutures or left open to heal.

Potential disabilities and complications: Zero to minimal long-term complications.

Surgery: Partial glossectomy (hemiglossectomy)

Description: Removal of up to half of the tongue muscle under general anesthesia, usually through the mouth. Recommended for T2, T3, or T4 cancers. Hospital stay is up to a week.

Reconstruction: Depending on the amount of tongue muscle removed, either closure with sutures or a skin graft or flap.

Potential disabilities and complications: Range is from minimal speech difficulties to significant speech and swallowing dysfunction. This usually is improved with speech therapy and continued practice. Temporary tracheostomy is often required.

Surgery: Near-total or total glossectomy
Description: Removal of all or most of the tongue. Reserved for very advanced cancers that allow few or no other options. Hospital stay is a week to ten days.
Reconstruction: Tongue muscle is replaced with a flap of muscle taken from either the chest or abdomen.
Potential disabilities and complications: Extensive speech and swallowing disruption. Some improvement will occur with practice and therapy. Some people will never eat normally and require a permanent feeding tube. A tracheostomy tube is usually required as well but is usually temporary.

Mandible (lower jaw bone)
Surgery: Marginal mandibulectomy
Description: If cancer is close to the mandible but has not invaded it, a portion of mandible closest to the tumor is removed, usually including some teeth. This does not disrupt the shape of the jaw. This is also done through the mouth. Hospital stay ranges from several days to over a week.
Reconstruction: If the tumor is small and on the top of the mandible, near the teeth, the soft tissues can usually be closed without any flap or graft. For larger tumors, a skin graft or flap is usually required. Any teeth taken out will usually be replaced by a denture after healing has occurred.
Potential disabilities and complications: Numbness of the lower lip and gums; gum pain; inability to wear dentures; slightly higher susceptibility to jaw fracture, both during the operation and afterwards; and bone infection.

Surgery: Segmental mandibulectomy
Description: Removal of an entire segment of the lower jaw. Done for larger tumors that invade or surround the mandible. Usually performed with major resection of tongue or floor of the mouth. Hospital stay, a week to ten days.
Reconstruction: If the bone is removed from the anterior (front) portion of the jaw, it must be replaced with bone. Small posterior defects may need to be replaced by bone.
Potential disabilities and complications: The same as for marginal mandibulectomy (above). Healing is slow, and a soft diet is required for six to eight weeks.

Hard Palate (hard portion of roof of the mouth)
Surgery: Hard palatectomy
Description: Removal of the hard palate, usually for tumors of the hard palate but sometimes as part of a maxillary sinus removal.
Reconstruction: Use of an obturator, a specialized denture that covers the hole created when the hard palate is removed. The obturator is cared for just like a regular denture. Hospital stay is usually two to five days.
Potential disabilities and complications: Speech and swallowing are impaired; the obturator helps with these problems.

Surgeries for Oropharynx Cancers

Tonsil
Surgery: Radical tonsillectomy
Description: Removal of the tonsil and surrounding tissue. Hospital stay is five to ten days.
Reconstruction: Depends on the depth of the resection; may require a flap for reconstruction.
Potential disabilities and complications: The wider the resection, the more likely it is that swallowing problems will arise; these are occasionally severe. Swallowing therapy may be required. Temporary tracheostomy may be required if flap is used.

Soft Palate (soft portion of roof of the mouth)
Surgery: Soft palatectomy
Description: Removal of some or all of the soft palate. Hospital stay, two to ten days.
Reconstruction: Usually none at the time of resection. An obturator (*see* hard palate surgery, above) is used for speech and swallowing after extensive removal of the palate. This is fashioned by a dental oncology specialist in the days and weeks following the surgery.
Potential disabilities and complications: Without an obturator, speech may have a nasal quality, and liquids may reflux into the nose. Tracheostomy is needed only with larger resections.

Posterior or Lateral Pharynx (back and side walls of the throat)

Surgery: Pharyngectomy

Description: Removal of the back or side walls of the throat. Sometimes done through the mouth or neck; sometimes requires splitting of the mandible and lower lip (that is, cutting the mandible in half and then plating it back together as with a jaw fracture). This is all done during the same operation. Hospital stay, seven to ten days.

Reconstruction: Skin graft or flap.

Potential disabilities and complications: Severe swallowing dysfunction, sometimes permanent; failure of the fracture to heal; a leak between the throat and the neck, called a *fistula,* which will heal with time and occasionally requires another operation; severe swelling of the larynx, which may respond to steroids. Tracheostomy is required but is usually temporary.

Base of the Tongue (rear portion of the tongue)

Surgery: Base of tongue resection

Description: Removal of part or all of the back part of the tongue. Hospital stay is usually two to ten days. This is typically done with robotic assistance.

Reconstruction: For early-stage cancers, simple closure is adequate. Higher-stage cancers usually require a muscle flap. (*See* pharyngectomy, above, for complications.)

Surgeries for Hypopharynx Cancers

Surgery: Partial pharyngectomy

Description: Removal of part of the pharynx, leaving the larynx intact. Reserved for very small cancers and usually done through the neck. Hospital stay, five to eight days.

Reconstruction: Closure with sutures.

Potential disabilities and complications: Swallowing dysfunction and speech problems, usually mild to moderate. A tracheostomy is often needed, which may be in place for several weeks to several months and occasionally is permanent.

Surgery: Total laryngopharyngectomy

Description: Removal of much or all of the pharynx and larynx.

Performed for advanced T3 and T4 hypopharyngeal cancers or those that have not responded to radiation therapy. Hospital stay, six to ten days.

Reconstruction: Typically requires a skin or muscle flap.

Potential disabilities and complications: Loss of ability to speak and swallow, which requires therapy. (*See* chapter 4 for a discussion of alternative speech methods.) A permanent breathing hole (stoma) in the lower neck, which does not permit a sense of smell. Major complications include a fistula, or leak, at the incision site. (*See also* laryngectomy, below.)

Surgeries on the Larynx

Glottis

Surgery: Micro-excision of laryngeal carcinoma

Description: With either a laser or scalpel, T1 and some T2 cancers of the vocal cords can be removed with the aid of a microscope. This is done either as an outpatient procedure or with an overnight hospital stay.

Reconstruction: None.

Potential disabilities and complications: Vocal quality may be permanently reduced if the resection is extensive. In rare cases, teeth may be chipped. In extremely rare cases, the laser can cause a fire in the airway, causing burns to the trachea.

Surgery: Vertical partial laryngectomy

Description: Removal of one vocal cord and part of the laryngeal cartilage (Adam's apple). Used for T1 and T2 glottic cancers, even if radiation has failed. Hospital stay, five to ten days; recovery, several weeks.

Reconstruction: Muscle flaps to replace the cord, rotated at the time of surgery.

Potential disabilities and complications: Severe difficulty swallowing, which requires further surgery. Hoarseness or somewhat breathy voice quality. Tracheostomy required; in rare cases where swelling does not go down, tracheostomy is permanent.

Supraglottis
Surgery: Supraglottic laryngectomy
Description: Removal of the false vocal cords and epiglottis. The true vocal cords remain intact. Used for previously untreated early-stage cancers. Hospital stay, five to ten days.
Reconstruction: Closure with sutures.
Potential disabilities and complications: Temporary tracheostomy; in rare cases, permanent. Aspiration of food and liquids into the lungs; most patients need therapy to learn how to eat safely. In less than 5 percent of cases, a permanent feeding tube is required.

Larynx
Surgery: Total laryngectomy
Description: Total removal of the voice box for advanced cancers of the larynx. May require removal of the thyroid gland or lymph nodes if the cancer has spread there. Also involves placement of a temporary feeding tube through the nose and into the stomach, to allow liquid tube feedings while the wound heals. Hospital stay is usually five to ten days.
Reconstruction: With the larynx removed, the trachea (breathing tube) is sewn directly to the skin of the lower neck, creating a stoma (hole) for breathing. The esophagus (formerly attached to the larynx) is sewn to the back of the tongue, creating a tube from the mouth to the stomach.
Potential disabilities and complications: Patients must relearn to swallow and speak. The stoma does not permit a sense of smell. Major complications include fistula (leak) through the incision.

Surgeries for Paranasal Sinus Cancers

Nasal Cavity (space from the nostrils to the back part of the nose-nasopharynx)
Surgery: Endoscopic resection
Description: For benign tumors and biopsies, an endoscope, an instrument that allows the surgeon to see areas too inaccessible through other means, can sometimes be used to facilitate removal of nasal or sinus lesions. This is usually done in the office or as an outpatient procedure.

Reconstruction: None.
Potential disabilities and complications: In very rare cases, the procedure can injure the optic nerve and cause blindness on the operated side.

Maxillary Sinus
Surgery: Maxillectomy (cheekbone and sinus)
Description: Removal of the maxillary sinus; necessary for most maxillary sinus cancers. Requires an incision either on the side of the nose or under the upper lip. Sometimes involves removing part of the roof of the mouth. Hospital stay is usually three to seven days.
Reconstruction: Use of an obturator (*See* hard palatectomy, above). A skin graft may be necessary to line the inside of the cavity.
Potential disabilities and complications: Facial numbness; facial disfigurement, requiring reconstructive surgery later on.

Ethmoid Sinus
Surgery: Ethmoidectomy, often with craniofacial resection
Description: Removal of ethmoid sinus, performed for most ethmoid sinus cancers. May involve removal of part of the cribriform plate in a procedure called a *craniofacial resection*. May also require removal of part of the covering of the brain (the dura), if this appears or proves cancerous. The dura can be patched at the time of surgery. Hospital stay is usually five to seven days.
Reconstruction: A local flap of tissue is used to rebuild the roof of the nose, thus separating the nasal cavity from the brain. This is done during the cancer surgery.
Potential disabilities or complications: The cerebrospinal fluid (CSF) covering the brain may leak from the nose; a drain, or spinal tap, is usually placed into the spinal canal during surgery so that the leak will stop and can seal over. CSF can become infected, causing meningitis, which is treated with antibiotics. In rare cases, swelling of the brain can cause headache or even a coma. Scarring can usually be well hidden.

Eyeball

Surgery: Orbital exenteration

Description: When the eyeball or any contents of the eye socket are cancerous, the eye may need to be removed. Hospital stay is usually three to seven days.

Reconstruction: Prosthetics specialists will create a very realistic looking eye, which will be fixed with special glue or attached to implanted magnets and pegs. Sometimes a skin or flap is used to reconstruct the area around the eye.

Potential disabilities and complications: Loss of depth perception, which requires both eyes working together. Most patients accommodate well over time without any specific therapy.

Surgeries for Salivary Gland Tumors

Parotid Gland

Surgery: Parotidectomy

Description: The parotid gland has two lobes, one superficial and one deep; these are separated by the nerve that controls the facial muscles. If the tumor is in the deep lobe then the entire parotid may need to be removed. The incision follows the crease in front of the ear, then curves around the earlobe and into the upper neck. Hospital stay is usually overnight.

Reconstruction: None, except in the case of permanent facial nerve paralysis. Nerve grafting may be done at the time of the operation if the facial nerve is removed. Reconstruction can improve facial dropping and eye closure.

Potential disabilities and complications: Injury to the facial nerve can weaken or paralyze facial muscles on one side of the face. Facial movement will usually return within several weeks or months. Other complications include: numbness of the earlobe, which can be permanent; hollowness of the cheek where the parotid gland was removed; drainage of saliva through the incision. Removal of the parotid gland can also cause nerves that stimulate saliva to grow into the sweat glands of the cheek skin, causing facial sweating. This is called *Frey's syndrome*. It is not a major problem, and it often responds to medication such as Botox injections, or even antiperspirants.

Submandibular Gland
Surgery: Submandibular gland excision
Description: Removal of the submandibular salivary gland, using an incision under the jawline. Usually an outpatient procedure.
Reconstruction: None.
Potential disabilities and complications: A slight hollowing and sharpening of the jaw line. Risk to certain nerves and their related functions, especially the nerves of the tongue and the lower lip.

Surgeries for Neck Tumors
Surgery: Selective, or modified, neck dissection
Description: Removal of lymph nodes along the jugular vein and under the jaw. Recommended for N0, N1, and selected N2 cancers in the neck. The submandibular gland is also removed, if nearby nodes are at risk of metastasis. Usually this is done in combination with other operations to the mouth and throat as listed above. When it is done alone, the hospital stay is two to four days.
Reconstruction: None. The incision follows a natural skin crease whenever possible.
Potential disabilities and complications: The neck is thinner at the site of the surgery, but this causes no functional impairment. Numbness of the skin of the neck, which usually gets better over six to twelve months. Nerves of the neck are potentially at risk, along with the functions they support. These include the nerve to the lower lip, nerves to the tongue, the nerve to the vocal cord, and the nerve to the shoulder. Physical therapy is often prescribed to improve shoulder function postoperatively.

Surgery: Radical neck dissection
Description: This takes the selective neck dissection further, removing nodes, the sternocleidomastoid muscle, the large neck muscle that runs from behind the ear to the clavicle, the spinal accessory nerve (which supports shoulder movement), and the internal jugular vein. This procedure is used for many N2A and N3 cancers. Hospital stay is usually three to five days when done alone.
Reconstruction: Usually none.

Potential disabilities and complications: Same as for selective neck dissection, with the addition of shoulder dysfunction and more pronounced thinning of the neck. Risks to the nerves mentioned above are slightly higher.

Common Reconstructive Surgeries

Surgery: Pectoralis major myocutaneous (large chest muscle under the breast) flap

Description: Use of chest muscle and overlying skin to reconstruct surgically removed muscle, especially to the tongue. Hospital stay is usually six to ten days.

Reconstruction: The area from which the muscle and skin are taken is closed. Occasionally, if a large amount of skin has been removed with the pectoralis muscle, a skin graft will be necessary.

Potential disabilities and complications: Mild weakness of the shoulder associated with certain types of movement. Usually fairly subtle. Thinning and scarring of the chest, from removal of the flap.

Surgery: Radial forearm free flap

Description: Skin and underlying soft tissue, including fat, are taken along with blood vessels (radial artery and veins). This thin, pliable flap is frequently used for the floor of the mouth. Hospital stay is usually five to eight days.

Reconstruction: The area from which the flap is taken is usually repaired with a skin graft taken from the thigh.

Potential disabilities and complications: Temporary discomfort; temporarily limited range of hand and wrist motion.

Surgery: Fibula (the non-weight-bearing bone of the lower leg) free flap

Description: The fibula (not the tibia or shinbone) is removed and used to reconstruct the jaw. Overlying skin is often used to reconstruct soft tissue in the mouth. Hospital stay is usually seven to eleven days.

Reconstruction: If only bone is removed, the incision is simply closed. If skin is also removed, a skin graft is used.

Appendix

Potential disabilities and complications: Temporary discomfort and temporary inability to bear full weight on the leg for one to three weeks.

Surgery: Anterior lateral thigh flap (skin and muscle from the thigh)
Description: The skin and one of the four quadriceps muscles are removed and used to reconstruct the soft tissue defects. Overlying skin is often used to reconstruct soft tissue in the mouth or neck. Hospital stay is usually five to seven days.
Reconstruction: In many cases the incision is simply closed. If the closure is too tight to safely close together, a skin graft is used.
Potential disabilities and complications: Temporary discomfort and temporary inability to bear full weight on the leg for one to three weeks.

Surgery: Rectus abdominus free flap
Description: Removal of an abdominal muscle to help reconstruct a large area of soft tissue. Hospital stay is usually six to nine days.
Reconstruction: The wound is closed.
Potential disabilities and complications: Temporary discomfort. Possible weakness or hernia of the abdominal wall.

Surgery: Split thickness skin graft
Description: A very thin, partial layer of skin is harvested, usually from the thigh. This kind of graft is used to resurface areas where bulk is not needed. Hospital stay is dictated by the other procedures performed.
Reconstruction: None.
Potential disabilities and complications: The area from which the skin graft is taken sometimes has a different color than adjacent skin.

Resources

American Academy of Hospice and Palliative Medicine

4700 West Lake Avenue
Glenview, IL 60025
Phone: (847) 375-4712
www.aahpm.org

American Academy of Otolaryngology— Head and Neck Surgery

1650 Diagonal Road
Alexandria, VA 22314
Phone: (703) 836-4444
www.entnet.org

American Cancer Society

15999 Clifton Road NE
Atlanta, GA 30329
Phone: (800) 227-2345
www.cancer.org

American Head and Neck Society

11300 West Olympic Boulevard, Suite 600
Los Angeles, CA 90064
Phone: (310) 437-0559
www.ahns.info

Association of Oncology Social Workers
100 North 20th Street, Suite 400
Philadelphia, PA 19103
Phone: (215) 599-6093
www.aosw.org

CancerCare Inc.
275 7th Avenue
New York, NY 10001
Phone: (800) 813-HOPE
www.cancercare.org

Hospice and Palliative Nurses Associaton
One Penn Center West, Suite 229
Pittsburgh, PA 15276
Phone: (412) 787-9301
www.hpna.org

National Association for Home Care and Hospice
228 Seventh Street SE
Washington, DC 20003
Phone: (202) 546-4759
www.nahc.org

National Hospice Organization and Palliative Care
1731 King Street, Suite 100
Alexandria, VA 22314
Phone: (703) 837-1500
www.nhpco.org

**Society of Otorhinolaryngology and
Head-Neck Nurses**
207 Downing Street
New Smyrna Beach, FL 32168
Phone: (386) 428-1695
www.sohnnurse.com

Support for People with Oral and Head and Neck Cancer

P.O. Box 53
Locust Valley, NY 11560
Phone: (800) 377-0928
www.spohnc.org

Glossary

A

acinic cell carcinoma: A malignant tumor of salivary glands occurring most commonly in the parotid gland.

adenocarcinoma: A malignant neoplasm of epithelial cells in glandular or glandlike pattern.

adenoid: Lymph tissue similar to tonsils located in the throat behind the nasal cavity, often referred to as the pharyngeal tonsil.

adenoid cystic carcinoma: A malignant neoplasm often occurring in the salivary glands with a proclivity to involve nerves.

adjuvant chemotherapy: Chemotherapy used with another treatment modality to increase effectiveness of treatment.

adjuvant radiation: Radiation used with another treatment modality (usually surgery) to increase effectiveness of treatment.

ameloblastoma: A nonmalignant tumor that arises from dental structures that has a proclivity for local recurrence.

American Joint Commission on Cancer: Commission dedicated to appropriate staging of cancer.

anaplastic thyroid cancer: An aggressive malignant neoplasm of the thyroid gland.

anaplastologist: Specialist who makes replacement prostheses for eyes, ears, and other body parts.

anesthesiologist: A physician who specializes in the administration of anesthesia.

artery: Blood vessel that carries oxygenated blood to the body.

153

aspiration: The inhalation of liquid, food, or other material into the windpipe and lungs.

B

barium swallow: A study in which a radiopaque suspension is swallowed for X-ray visualization of the gastrointestinal tract.

benign: Not cancerous or malignant.

biopsy: Surgical removal of part or all of a mass or organ for diagnostic purposes.

bladder: Organ that collects urine from the kidneys.

boughies: Cylindrical, flexible instruments of various diameters used to dilate the esophagus.

brachytherapy: Radiotherapy in which the source of irradiation is placed close to the surface of the skin or within the body.

C

candida albicans: A fungus that is normally part of the gastrointestinal tract, but which may cause infection.

cardiologist: Physician who specializes in diseases of the heart.

cautery: Heating device used to stop bleeding in the operating room.

cellulitis: Inflammation of the skin.

central venous catheter: A catheter placed in one of the central veins (large veins near the heart) for delivery of intravenous medication or nutrients.

cerebral spinal fluid (CSF): Fluid surrounding the brain and spinal cord.

chemotherapy: Treatment of disease by means of chemical substances or drugs.

computer assisted tomography (CT scan): A special X-ray used to evaluate organs and tissues within the body.

cyst: Noncancerous growth, usually filled with fluid.

D

dental oncologist: A specialist who cares for the teeth of patients with cancer to prevent dental complications from treatment and fabricates prosthetics to rehabilitate swallowing and speech.

dura: Protective covering of the brain and spinal cord.

Glossary

E

echocardiogram: Diagnostic test using ultrasound to evaluate the heart.

electrocardiogram: An electrical tracing of the heart's rhythm.

electrolarynx: A handheld battery-operated device that is used to create mechanical speech after removal of the voice box.

endocrinologist: A physician specializing in the secreting glands within the body.

ENT doctor: A physician, also known as an *otolaryngologist,* who specializes in diseases of the ears, nose, and throat.

epiglottis: A leaf-shaped cartilage structure covered with mucosa just above the larynx that assists in prevention of liquid or food entering the voice box.

Epstein-Barr virus: A virus implicated in the cause of nasopharyngeal carcinoma.

erythroplakia: A red, velvety plaque-like patch of mucous membrane that may represent malignant change.

esophageal speech: A technique of swallowing air and then belching the air to form words.

esophagus: The portion of the digestive tract between the throat and stomach.

esthesioneuroblastoma: A cancer arising from the olfactory nerves in the top of the nasal cavity.

eustachian tube: A tube leading from the middle ear to the nasopharynx.

external beam radiation: Radiotherapy in which irradiation is delivered from a source outside the body.

extirpation: Surgical removal of diseased tissue.

F

facial nerve: The nerve that controls the muscles of facial expression.

false vocal cords: Paired structures within the voice box just below the true vocal cords.

fibula: The outer and smaller, non-weight-bearing bone of the lower leg.

fine needle aspiration (FNA): Needle biopsy of tissue or organ for diagnostic purposes.

flap: Surgical creation of a segment of tissue with intact blood supply for movement to another area of the body.

Foley catheter: Plastic tube inserted into the bladder through the urethra to empty the bladder.

follicular thyroid cancer: Malignant neoplasm of the thyroid gland arising from follicular cells within the gland.

free flap: A segment of tissue transferred to another part of the body with surgical microvascular connection of the blood vessels.

Frey's syndrome: A complication that can occur after surgical removal of the parotid gland characterized by sweating of the cheek skin when eating. Also known as *gustatory sweating.*

frozen section: A technique of freezing tissue for examination under the microscope, usually in an attempt to determine presence or absence of diseased tissue such as cancer.

G

gastroenterologist: A physician who specializes in diseases of the gastrointestinal tract.

gastroesophageal reflux: Regurgitation of stomach contents into the esophagus, commonly referred to as heartburn.

gastrostomy tube: A tube surgically placed through the skin into the stomach to deliver nutrients.

general anesthesia: Anesthesia used during surgery causing the patient to sleep.

gingivitis: Inflammation of the gums.

glottis: Voice box, especially the true vocal cords.

grade: Microscopic characterization of the cellular activity of a malignancy usually into high and low.

graft: An unattached portion of tissue for transplantation.

H

head/neck surgical oncologist: Surgeon who specializes in the care of patients with cancers of the head and neck.

home health nurse: Nurse who specializes in the care of patients at home.

Glossary

hospice: An institution that provides supportive and palliative care for dying patients.

human papillomavirus (HPV): A virus implicated in causing disease especially cancer of the tonsil and base of tongue.

hyperbaric oxygen (HBO): Treatment using high-pressure oxygen in a chamber to heal or prevent disease often resulting from irradiation.

hyperthyroidism: A disease in which the thyroid gland produces too much thyroid hormone.

hypoglossal nerve: Nerve that controls the movement of the tongue.

hypothyroidism: A disease in which the thyroid gland does not produce enough thyroid hormone.

I

immunotherapy: Drugs that alter the body's immune cells to enhance their ability to kill cancer cells.

informed consent: A process in which a patient or guardian authorized specific treatment.

institutional review board (IRB): An organization composed of physicians and others governing the implementation of studies to ensure protection of patient rights and safety.

intensive care unit (ICU): Hospital area where acutely ill patients go to recover after major surgery.

internal jugular vein: Large vein that carries blood from the head and neck to the heart.

intravenous catheter (IV): A small catheter placed into a vein to deliver intravenous fluid, medication, chemical substances, or nutrients.

inverted papilloma: A benign tumor of the nose or sinuses that is locally destructive and in 10 percent of cases may harbor malignancy.

L

larynx: Voice box.

leukoplakia: White plaque-like patches of mucosa that may be precancerous.

lidocaine: Medication used to anesthetize (numb) tissue.

lingual nerve: Nerve that controls sensation to the tongue.

living will: Document explaining a patient's wishes for the use of life-support measures in case he or she is incapacitated.

local anesthesia: Injection of medicine into an area, numbing it to pain so a surgeon can perform local surgery.

lymph node: Small bean-shaped structures throughout the body that fight infection.

lymphatics: Channels throughout the body that transport lymph fluid.

lymphoepithelial cancer: A malignancy of epithelial cell origin involving lymphoid tissues of the tonsils and nasopharynx.

lymphoma: Malignant neoplasm of lymph tissue.

M

magnetic resonance imaging (MRI): Highly specialized X-ray using electrons to take detailed pictures of organs and tissues.

malignant: A neoplasm capable of local invasion, destructive growth, and metastasis.

mandible: Lower jaw bone.

marginal mandibulectomy: Partial removal of lower jaw bone.

maxilla: Upper jaw bone.

maxillectomy: Surgical removal of upper jaw bone.

medical oncologist: Nonsurgeon physician who specializes in the treatment of patients with cancer.

medullary thyroid cancer: Type of cancer of the thyroid gland.

melanin: Dark brown to black pigment of skin.

melanoma: Malignant neoplasm of skin arising from cells that produce melanin.

melatonin: Hormone produced by the pineal gland.

metastasis: The spread of malignant cells to different parts of the body.

minor salivary glands: Microscopic glands numbering between 600 to 1000 that line the tongue, lips, palate, throat, nose, and sinuses.

mixed tumor: The most common tumor of the salivary glands occurring most commonly in the parotid gland. Although benign, a small percentage may convert to malignancy. Also known as *pleomorphic adenoma.*

modified neck dissection: Surgical procedure to remove the lymph nodes from the neck in which the technique is modified to spare one or more of the following structures: the spinal accessory nerve, the sternocleidomastoid muscle, or the internal jugular.

mucoepidermoid carcinoma: Most common malignant tumor of the salivary glands.

mucositis: Inflammation of the mucosa of the mouth and throat due to radiation therapy or chemotherapy, resulting in painful sores.

myotomy: Surgical division of muscle.

N

narcotic: A potent drug used to treat pain.

nasogastric tube: Tube that passes through the nose into the stomach used for decompressing the stomach or for feeding.

nasopharynx: Anatomic area of the throat located directly behind the nose.

neck dissection: Surgical procedure to remove the lymph nodes from the neck.

O

obturator: Denture-like prosthesis used to fill the space between the mouth and nose.

olfactory nerve: Nerves that control smell, located at the top of the nasal cavity.

oncologist: Physician who specializes in the care of patients with cancer.

organ preservation: Treatment strategy aimed at preserving an important organ involved with cancer.

osteoradionecrosis: Bone tissue death due to inadequate blood supply from irradiation.

otolaryngologist: Physician who specializes in diseases of the ear, nose, and throat. Also known as an *ENT doctor.*

P

palliation: Treatment strategy aimed at providing relief of symptoms from incurable cancer.

papillary thyroid cancer: Most common type of malignant tumor of the thyroid gland.

parotid gland: Largest of the salivary glands located in the cheeks just in front of and underneath the ears.

partial laryngectomy: Partial removal of the voice box.

pathologist: A physician who specializes in anatomical and microscopic examination of tissue to determine cause of disease.

patient-controlled-analgesia (PCA): Device used after surgery that allows the patients to give themselves narcotic pain medicine.

pectoralis major myocutaneous flap: Tissue including muscle and skin from the chest often used to reconstruct the areas in the head and neck after tumor removal.

pharynx: Throat.

pituitary gland: A gland located near the brain responsible for hormonal regulation.

placebo effect: When a sugar pill or inactive medicine is given to a person without their knowledge that it is an inactive medicine, and they get better.

platelets: Components circulating in the bloodstream that assist with blood clotting.

pleomorphic adenoma: The most common tumor of the salivary glands occurring most commonly in the parotid gland. Although benign, a small percentage may convert to malignancy. Also known as a *mixed tumor*.

polyp: Inflammatory mass of swollen mucosa.

primary: Relating to the first growth or development of a tumor.

prosthetics: Synthetic material used to replace tissue.

prosthodontist: A specialist in the use of prosthetic medical material.

pulse oximeter: Machine that continuously measures the level of oxygenation in the blood through a small device attached to a fingertip or earlobe.

R

Glossary

radial forearm flap: A flap of tissue and sometimes a portion of the radius bone from the forearm used to reconstruct surgical defects.

radiation oncologist: A physician who specializes in the use of irradiation to treat disease, especially malignant tumors.

radiation therapy: The use of irradiation to treat disease.

radical neck dissection: Surgical removal of the lymph nodes in the neck along with the spinal accessory nerve, internal jugular vein, and sternocleidomastoid muscle.

radiologist: Physician trained to perform and interpret X-ray studies.

radius: The outer of the two bones in the forearm.

respiratory therapist: A health-care worker with formal training in diseases of the lungs who administers treatments to hospitalized patients with lung ailments.

S

salivary glands: Glands located in the head and neck responsible for production of saliva.

sarcoma: Malignant tumor that arises from connective tissue, muscle, bone, or cartilage.

scapula: Shoulder-blade bone.

second primary: A new tumor unrelated to an original tumor, in contrast to recurrent tumor or metastasis.

simulation: The planning phase for treatment with irradiation.

sinuses (ethmoid, frontal, maxillary, and sphenoid): Paired bony cavities lined by mucous membranes contiguous with the nasal cavity.

skin graft: Skin harvested from another part of the body to resurface another area of the body.

speech pathologist: Specialist trained to help with speech and swallowing disorders.

spinal accessory nerve: Nerve located in the neck controlling movement of the trapezius muscle. Injury to this nerve can result in difficulty elevating the shoulder.

squamous cell carcinoma: Malignant neoplasm arising from epithelial cells, and the most common malignant tumor of the head and neck.

staging: Process of how advanced a malignant neoplasm is determined.

sternocleidomastoid muscle: Large muscle within the neck extending from behind the ear to the middle of the base of the neck.

stoma: Opening between the skin and windpipe.

subglottis: Area of the airway located just below the vocal cords.

sublingual gland: Salivary gland located on the inside of the mouth between the side of the tongue and the jaw bone.

submandibular gland: Salivary gland located just below and near the jaw bone.

supraglottic laryngectomy: Removal of the top portion of the voice box.

supraglottis: Area of the airway located just above the vocal cords.

T

targeted therapy: The use of drugs that very specifically affect a particular gene or protein designed to slow or halt cancer cell growth.

TNM system: A staging system used to assess how advanced a neoplasm is including size of the tumor, presence of spread to lymph nodes, and metastasis.

thrush: Fungal infection of the mouth or throat.

thyroid gland: Gland in the neck under the Adam's apple that secretes thyroid hormone.

thyroid hormone: Hormone secreted by the thyroid gland that helps regulate the body's metabolism.

thyroid stimulating hormone: Hormone secreted by the pituitary gland that regulates the production of thyroid hormone.

thyroidectomy: Surgical removal of the thyroid gland.

total laryngectomy: Surgical removal of the entire voice box.

Glossary

tracheoesophageal puncture: A surgical communication created between the trachea (windpipe) and esophagus where a valve is placed so that air can be shunted to the esophagus and then belched to form speech.

tracheostomy: Surgical creation of a hole in the windpipe to assist with breathing.

trapezius muscle: Large muscle on the back of the neck, shoulder, and upper back that assists with elevation of the shoulder.

trismus: Limited opening of the jaws.

tumor: Swelling or mass of tissue synonymous with neoplasm.

U

ultrasound: Diagnostic test that uses sound waves to evaluate tissues and organs.

Union for International Cancer Control: International organization for staging cancer.

V

vocal cords: Paired cords of tissue within the voice box that vibrate to produce speech.

X

xerostomia: Dry mouth.

INDEX

Index

Index

Index

hot flashes, 78
human papillomavirus (HPV), 6,
    14, 18, 19, 33, 88, 106
    staging HPV oropharynx can-
    cers, 33
hydration, 60, 71
    after radiation therapy, 59
hydrazine, 4
hydrocodone, 99
hydromorphone, 99
hyoid bone, 9, 14
hyperbaric oxygen (HBO)
    treatments, 63
hypopharynx, 8, 30, 31, 87, 92

I

ibuprofen, 47, 73, 100
imaging studies, 26, 32, 35, 39,
    83, 84, 85
immune deficiency, 7
immune system, 6, 80, 104
immunotherapy, 66, 69, 80, 81
    overview, 80, 81
    receiving, 81
    side effects, 81
incision drainage, 46, 47
infections, 8, 10, 16, 20, 32, 47,
    62, 73, 75, 80
    after chemotherapy, 72
    after surgery, 46
    at incision site, 46, 47
    signs of, 46, 47
infertility, 77, 78
inflammation, 62, 100
informed consent, 116, 118
infusions of chemotherapy, 68
initial biopsy, 25
initial examination, 23
institutional review board (IRB),
    115, 116
insurance considerations, 133

intensity-modulated radiation
    therapy (IMRT), 57
intensive care unit (ICU), 46
internal jugular vein, 42, 145
internal radiation therapy, 57, 89
    see also brachytherapy
intravenous IV delivery of
    targeted therapy, 79
intravenous IV line, 39, 67
investigator-initiated trials, 114
iodine contrast material, 27
    allergic reaction, 27
iron supplements, 72
irregular menstrual periods, 78
isopropyl exposure, 7
IV fluids, 71

J

jaw,
    decreased opening, 65
jaw bone, 14, 47, 62, 89, 140
jaw joint, 65

K

keratin, 125
kidneys, 5, 76, 81
    damage due to tobacco use,
    4

L

laboratory testing, 116
laryngeal cartilage, 141
    see also Adam's apple
larynx, 1, 9, 19, 23, 24, 25, 30,
    31, 84, 87, 88, 89
    compartments, 10
    function abnormalities, 23
    operations on the larynx,
    141, 142
    removal, 51
    swelling, 140
    swelling after radiation
    therapy, 65

171

Index

Index

Index

red patches in mouth or throat, 19
redness of skin, 47
 after surgery, 46
referred pain, 21
regional lymph nodes, 31
rehabilitation, 124
rehabilitation after radiation therapy, 60
rehabilitation after surgery, 49, 51
relaxation techniques, 71, 92, 95, 108
reproductive specialist, 78
research studies, 113
respiratory illnesses, 126
respiratory system, 10
rhahdomyosarcoma, 16
ringing in ears, 74
robotic surgery, 45, 140
roof of mouth, 8, 16, 139, 143
 see also hard palate

S
saliva, 42, 56, 59, 61
salivary gland, 12, 14, 19, 27, 42, 59, 61, 87, 90, 91
 damage due to tobacco use, 4
 function, 59
 suspicious lumps, 24
 tumors, 30
salivary gland cancers, 1, 19, 33
 most common, 15
salivary gland tumors, 14, 15
salivary substitutes, 59
sarcomas, 16, 29, 91
 staging, 34, 35
 types, 16
second opinions, 35, 110
secondary cancer formation, 65

secondary smoke, 126
sedatives, 55
segmental mandibulectomy, 138
selective neck dissection, 42, 145
sense of smell, 17, 142
sense of taste, 85
septum, 20
sexual and reproductive changes, after chemotherapy, 77, 78
sexual function, 77
sexual health, 133
sexual organs, 77
sexually transmitted virus, 6
shinbone, 146
shortness of breath, 76, 81
shoulder weakness, 51, 145, 146
side effects of immunotherapy, 81
 management of treatment-related, 132
side effects of chemotherapy, 68–78
side effects of radiation therapy
 long-term, 58, 59
 short-term, 58, 59
side effects of surgery, 42–46
single therapies, 86
sinus, sinuses,
 damage due to tobacco use, 4
sinus infections, 12
sinus lesions, 142
sinus tumors, 12, 21
sinuses, 1, 11, 12, 33, 61, 73
 after radiation therapy, 61
skin, 17, 73, 81
skin cancers, 7, 8, 14, 33
skin care, 64
skin changes, 76

Index

Index

About the Authors

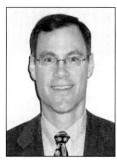

William Lydiatt, M.D., is a board-certified otolaryngologist—a head and neck surgeon. He practices oncology surgery at Nebraska Methodist Hospital in Omaha, Nebraska. He also teaches and performs research at the Creighton University School of Medicine. His research interests include improving the quality of life for head and neck cancer patients and the prevention of depression, using education and wellness.

Dr. Lydiatt received his undergraduate degree in biology from Stanford University, then his medical degree and residency training in otolaryngology—head and neck surgery—from the University of Nebraska. He also completed a two-year fellowship in head and neck surgical oncology at Memorial Sloan-Kettering Cancer Center in New York City.

Dr. Lydiatt is a fellow of the American College of Surgeons, American Board of Otolaryngology–Head and Neck Surgery, and American Head and Neck Society. He is the vice chair of the American Joint Commission on Cancer Staging Subcommittee for head and neck cancer staging; he is a reviewer for six specialty journals. Dr. Lydiatt has authored more than one hundred scientific publications and delivered hundreds of local, national, and international presentations on head and neck cancer. He enjoys teaching residents, medical students, physician assistants, and other medical trainees.

Dr. Lydiatt and his wife, Kathy, have three children—Max, Joe, and Samantha. Dr. Lydiatt may be reached through Omaha's Methodist Hospital website: **www.bestcare.org.**

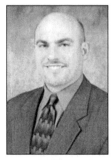

Perry Johnson, M.D., F.A.C.S., is a professor and chief of the division of plastic and reconstructive surgery at the University of Nebraska. Dr. Johnson is dually boarded in plastic surgery and otolaryngology by the American Board of Plastic Surgery and the American Board of Otolaryngology–Head and Neck Surgery, respectively. His areas of interest and expertise include head and neck cancer reconstruction, breast cancer reconstruction, and skin cancer reconstruction. Dr. Johnson's practice also focuses on plastic surgery of the breast, and aesthetic surgery, in particular rhinoplasty.

Dr. Johnson received a bachelor of arts in chemistry from the University of Kansas. He also received his medical degree from the University of Kansas. Following medical school, he completed a residency in otolaryngology–head and neck surgery at the University of Nebraska. He then completed an additional residency in plastic and reconstructive surgery at the University of Pittsburgh.

Dr. Johnson is a fellow of the American College of Surgery, the American Society of Plastic Surgery, the American Academy of Otolaryngology—Head and Neck Surgery, and multiple other professional organizations. He is one of the founders and former program director of the plastic surgery residency training program at the University of Nebraska. He remains active in the teaching of residents, medical students, physician assistants, and other medical trainees.

Dr. Johnson served on the editorial board of the Archives of Facial Plastic Surgery and serves on a number of professional medical committees. He has authored numerous scientific publications including books, book chapters, and medical journal articles and has given presentations on plastic surgery regionally, nationally, and internationally.

Dr. Johnson may be reached through his website: **www.surgeryvp.com**

Consumer Health Titles from Addicus Books

Visit our online catalog at www.AddicusBooks.com

To Order Books:
Visit us online at: www.AddicusBooks.com
Call toll free: (800) 888-4741

For discounts on bulk purchases, call our Special Sales
Department at (402) 330-7493.
Or email us at: info@Addicus Books.com

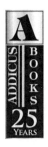

Addicus Books
P. O. Box 45327
Omaha, NE 68145

*Addicus Books is dedicated to publishing consumer health books
that comfort and educate.*